Disasters and Mass Casualty Incidents

Editor
Mauricio Lynn

Associate Editors
Howard Lieberman · Lior Lynn
Gerd Daniel Pust · Kenneth Stahl
Daniel Dante Yeh · Tanya Zakrison

Disasters and Mass Casualty Incidents

The Nuts and Bolts of Preparedness and Response to Protracted and Sudden Onset Emergencies

Second Edition

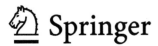 Springer

Editor
Mauricio Lynn
Miller School of Medicine
University of Miami
Miami, FL
USA

Associate Editors
Howard Lieberman
Miller School of Medicine
University of Miami Health System
Miami, FL
USA

Lior Lynn
Lynn Therapy
Pembroke Pines
FL
USA

Gerd Daniel Pust
Miller School of Medicine
University of Miami Health System
Miami, FL
USA

Kenneth Stahl
Miller School of Medicine
University of Miami Health System
Miami, FL
USA

Daniel Dante Yeh
Miller School of Medicine
University of Miami Health System
Miami, FL
USA

Tanya Zakrison
Miller School of Medicine
University of Miami Health System
Miami, FL
USA

ISBN 978-3-319-97360-9   ISBN 978-3-319-97361-6   (eBook)
https://doi.org/10.1007/978-3-319-97361-6

Library of Congress Control Number: 2018959150

This Springer imprint is published by the registered company Springer Nature Switzerland AG
The registered company address is: Gewerbestrasse 11, 6330 Cham, Switzerland

Preface

This manual is not meant to replace other "disaster books." It is designed to provide a simplified operational blueprint, for health care professionals and emergency managers, for planning the response and medical management during events with large number of sick and injured patients.

The first edition, *Mass Casualty Incidents: The Nuts and Bolts of Preparedness and Response for Acute Disasters"* published in 2016, dealt exclusively with events that are abrupt in nature.

This second edition expands its focus and includes preparations and response for insidious and protracted disasters as well.

Most of the information in this manual is derived from the Israeli experience in managing mass casualty events for almost 70 years. Some of this knowledge was adapted to Emergency Medical Services and medical centers in the United States and other countries.

Much of the material in this manual is based on the proficiency of many experts with whom I had the opportunity to work and learn. I would like to acknowledge some of my colleagues, partners, teachers, and friends, who through their wisdom and spirit helped me put together this manual (in alphabetical order):

Bruria Adini, Hani Bahouth, Dan Deckelbaum, Arieh Eldad, Zvi Feigenberg, Gila Heims, Asher Hirshberg, Jeffery Kashuk, Yoram Klein, Yoram Kluger, Guy Lin, Abdul Memom, Moshe Michelson, Nicholas Namias, Kobi Peleg, Dror Soffer, Michael Stein, Ilan Tur-Kaspa, Steve Williams.

Special thanks to my lovely wife Iris, who supports me since we met 34 years ago and has been an anchor in my life. My special love to our children Barak, Lior, and Royi, from whom I learned to respect other opinions, despite mine being always the right one.

This second edition is dedicated to my mother Paula, who encouraged me to do what I love, and to my father Shamariahu, who was always my role model. Let them both rest in peace.

Miami, FL, USA
Mauricio Lynn, MD, FACS

Contents

Contributors

Alex Canales Jackson Memorial Hospital, Miami Beach, FL, USA

Shabnam Hafiz, MD, MPH Ryder Trauma Center, Jackson Memorial Hospital, Department of Surgery, Miami, FL, USA

Asaf Kedar, MD Jackson Memorial Hospital, University of Miami Miller School of Medicine, DeWitt Daughtry Family Department of Surgery, Division of Trauma/Critical Care/Burns, Miami, FL, USA

Howard Lieberman, BSc, MSc, MD Jackson Memorial Hospital-Ryder Trauma-University of Miami, Department of Trauma and Acute Care Surgery/Surgical Care, Miami, FL, USA

Lior Lynn, MSEd Lynn Therapy, LLC, Pembroke Pines, FL, USA

Mauricio Lynn, MD, FACS University of Miami Miller School of Medicine, Jackson Memorial Hospital, Department of Surgery, Miami, FL, USA

Caleb J. Mentzer, DO Memorial Hermann Hospital, Department of Surgery, Division of Acute Care Surgery, University of Texas Health Science Center, Houston, TX, USA

Bradley S. Moffat, MD, MSc Jackson Memorial Hospital, Ryder Trauma Center, Miami, FL, USA

Henry Morgenstern Security Solutions International INC, Miami, FL, USA

Nicholas Namias, MD University of Miami Miller School of Medicine, Jackson Memorial Hospital, Department of Surgery, Miami, FL, USA

Gerd Daniel Pust, MD, FACS University of Miami/Jackson Memorial Hospital, The DeWitt Daughtry Family Department of Surgery, Miami, FL, USA

Alon D. Schwartz, MD Trauma and Acute Care Surgery, Shaare Zedek Medical Center, Department of General Surgery, Jerusalem, Israel

Hahn Soe-Lin, MD, MS Ryder Trauma Center, Jackson Memorial Hospital, Department of Surgery, Miami, FL, USA

Kenneth Stahl, MD University of Miami Miller School of Medicine, Jackson Memorial Hospital, Department of Surgery, Miami, FL, USA

D. Dante Yeh, MD Ryder Trauma Center, Department of Surgery, Miami, FL, USA

Lauren Zakaib, PsyS, MS Psychological Services, Broward County School District, Fort Lauderdale, FL, USA

Tanya L. Zakrison, MD University of Miami Miller School of Medicine, Jackson Memorial Hospital, Department of Surgery, Miami, FL, USA

Part I

Planning and Response to Sudden Mass Casualty Incidents

General Information

1

Mauricio Lynn

Introduction

This section will set up the stage for the entire book with the objective to better clarify its focus.

Planning to handle catastrophes should be according to the speed that the initial medical response requires to handle the increased number of patients, and the initial ratio between caregivers and patients.

From a medical perspective, the most difficult challenge is to respond to an event that occurred suddenly, without prior notice and with a large number of injured or contaminated patients. The Sarin gas attack in the Tokyo subway in 1995, where more than 5000 people were contaminated, the Madrid train bombings in 2004, with more than 2000 casualties and the Mass Shooting incident in Las Vegas in 2017, where more than 800 people were injured, are great examples of large-scale, unplanned mass casualty incidents.

Therefore, the definition and classification of disasters in this section is different than in other publications. It is the introduction of the concept of sudden mass casualty incident (SMCI).

Definitions

In other publications, disasters and mass casualty incidents (MCIs) are interchangeable concepts. Nevertheless, from a medical perspective, there is a need to separate the definitions, since almost all MCIs are 'disasters' for the community, but not all disasters are associated with MCIs.

M. Lynn
University of Miami Miller School of Medicine, Jackson Memorial Hospital,
Department of Surgery, Miami, FL, USA
e-mail: mlynn@med.miami.edu

© Springer Nature Switzerland AG 2019
M. Lynn et al. (eds.), *Disasters and Mass Casualty Incidents*,
https://doi.org/10.1007/978-3-319-97361-6_1

Disaster

- A disaster is a natural or man-made hazard resulting in significant physical damage or destruction, loss of life or drastic change to the environment (Fig. 1.1).
- From a medical perspective, a disaster may cause injuries, contamination or disease to people, or may be associated with only physical damage, without affecting the health of human beings.

Mass Casualty Incident (MCI)

A mass casualty incident (MCI) is an event where the number of patients temporarily exceeds the capability of the first responders at the scene or of the medical staff at the hospital to provide optimal care to all victims simultaneously.

A MCI is a 'temporary state of insufficiency' (Fig. 1.2).

- At the pre-hospital phase, the 'state of insufficiency' may be due to:
  - Insufficient *access* and *evacuation* routes for ambulances.
  - Insufficient number of *ambulances* and/or *helicopters* during the initial phase.
  - Insufficient number of *personnel* (drivers, paramedics, physicians (if applicable) during the first hours.
  - Insufficient amount of *equipment* and *supplies*.
- At the hospital phase, the 'state of insufficiency' may be due to:
  - Insufficient number of *personnel* (doctors, nurses, technicians, transporters, clerks, security guards) during the initial phase.
  - Insufficient *space* in the emergency department (ED) or intensive care unit(s).

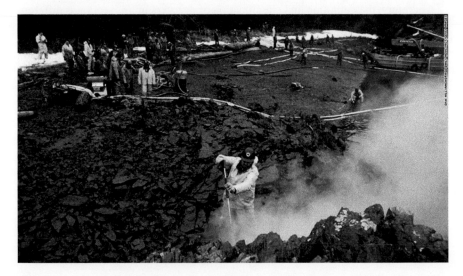

Fig. 1.1 Exxon oil spill, considered one of the largest ecological disasters in modern history, 1989

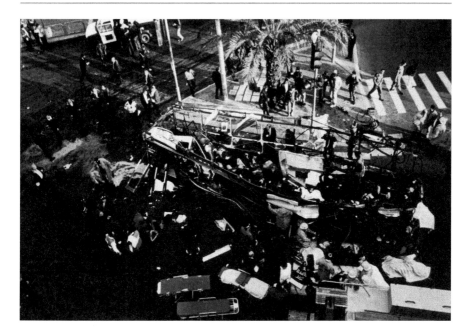

Fig. 1.2 Bus explosion by suicide bomber, Jerusalem, Israel, 2006

- Insufficient number of *operating rooms* available.
- Insufficient number of available *ventilators*.
- Insufficient amount of *supplies*.
- Insufficient number of *blood* units available for immediate use.

Even in countries where MCIs are common, there will always be a 'state of insufficiency' both at the pre-hospital and at the hospital.

The main objective of a well-written and detailed disaster plan combined with frequent live exercises and drills is to shorten the period of 'insufficiency'.

Classification

Disasters and catastrophes may be divided into two major categories, according to the initial medical response:

Progressive Disasters or Pre-planned Mass Gatherings

A progressive disaster may occur over a long period of time, such as days, weeks, months or even years.

From a medical perspective, the individuals inside the Chernobyl nuclear reactor did not survive the initial explosion, but up to these days, there is a higher incidence of thyroid cancer among those people exposed to the radiation (Fig. 1.3).

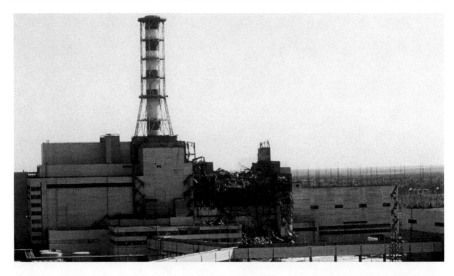

Fig. 1.3 Chernobyl nuclear reactor after the accident, 1986

Fig. 1.4 Patient with smallpox

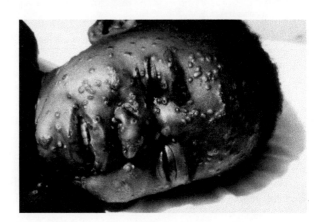

A typical progressive event is the slow spread of a biological agent (Fig. 1.4). The total number of infected patients may be enormous, but characteristically, not all arrive at *one* emergency department (ED) simultaneously. Sick patients will either go to their primary care physician first or to the closest ED.

Another good example of a progressive event is the slow evolution of a hurricane. Typically, the path of a major storm may be known for days before it makes landfall. Its slow progression allows for evacuation of populations at risk and deployment of emergency personnel and equipment prior to storm arrival.

The *medical response* for a progressive disaster should be in place *before* the event reaches its full magnitude.

Similar planning and response may be used for mass gatherings, such as major sporting events, concerts or air shows. In these situations, risk assessment is

performed, potential threats are analyzed and possible medical consequences are considered. According to the findings, all or fractions of the planned medical response may be deployed prior to the event:
- Ambulances
- Medical personnel
- Helicopters
- On-site decontamination facilities
- Pre-planned access and evacuation routes

Sudden Mass Casualty Incidents

A sudden mass casualty incidents (SMCI) may be a result of a train or plane crash, earthquake, explosion or mass shooting. The common theme of all these events is that they occur without prior warning. This fact results in a *'temporary state of insufficiency'*, described previously.

SMCIs may be of conventional nature, more commonly traumatic, blast and burn injuries, chemical exposure to hazardous materials or a radiological dispersal device (RDD), also known as 'dirty bomb'.

Unlike with progressive disasters, the *medical response* for SMCIs is initiated *after* the event has already reached its full magnitude. This circumstance presents as a major challenge for the first responders at the scene as well as for the hospitals that need to absorb and treat a large number of injured patients, with minimal time to prepare.

A large-scale SMCI (e.g. Madrid train bombing, mass shooting in Las Vegas, earthquakes) may overwhelm the medical resources of a city, its emergency medical services (EMS), medical centres, medical examiner and mortuaries. It is this type of incident that may require external help, from within the state, the country or international.

Epidemiology of Sudden Mass Casualty Incidents and Its Practical Applications

The main goal of the medical response to a sudden mass casualty incident (SMCI) is to *identify and manage the critical patients* in an attempt to save lives. For planning purposes, it is imperative to know the approximate number of severe or critical patients to expect after a SMCI. Therefore, it is important to learn the epidemiology of such events.

Examples of SMCIs include
- Explosions.
- Plane crashes.
- Train derailments.
- Earthquakes (Fig. 1.5).

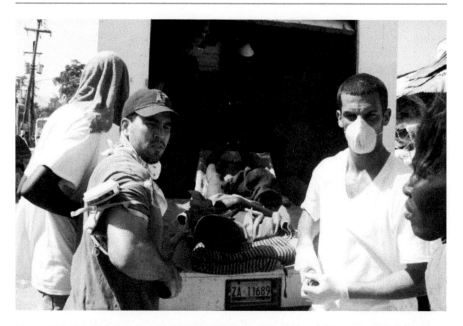

Fig. 1.5 Relief efforts, Haiti earthquake, 2010

Fig. 1.6 Volcanic
eruption, Hawaii, 2018

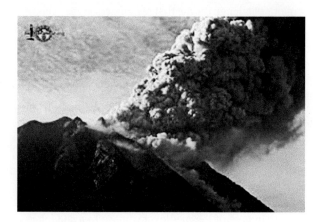

- Volcanic eruptions (Fig. 1.6).
- Mass shootings.
- Massive chemical contamination (Fig. 1.7).
- Radiological dispersal device (RDD) or 'dirty bomb'.

Regardless of the type of SMCI, the *vast majority* of the injured or contaminated patients will be walking wounded.

In all examples above, the number of critical patients, who require immediate attention, is low and rarely exceeds 20% of the total number of injured.

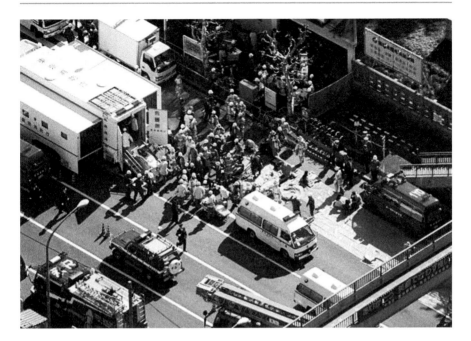

Fig. 1.7 Sarin gas attack, Tokyo, 1995

Planning for a MCI should focus on directing resources, such as personnel, equipment and supplies, to manage those few who are critically injured and/or contaminated and *salvageable*.

The concept of *'the greatest good for the greatest number' is a myth,* and it is not supported by any published literature regarding the severity of injuries in an urban SMCI.

Prehospital Planning and Response to Sudden Mass Casualty Incidents

Mauricio Lynn

Introduction

This section describes important topics of the planning of the response for the first responders, in particular the emergency medical services (EMS), to a sudden mass casualty incident (SMCI).

The section includes the prehospital phases of a sudden mass casualty incident (SMCI), discusses the limitations of deploying a scene incident command (SIC) and regional emergency operations center (REOC) for this type of events, stressing the importance of a coordinated communication system.

Finally, the section introduces a new concept such as "Save and Run" and discusses the pitfalls of patient tracking at the scene of the incident and the importance of patient tracking at the hospital.

Phases and Characteristics of Mass Casualty Incidents

All sudden mass casualty incidents (SMCIs) have common characteristics. It is important to be familiar with them as they will have a major impact on the prehospital as well as on the hospital planning of the response.

Chaos Phase

The initial minutes following any SMCI are known as the *chaos phase*. It is characterized by a lack of leadership, organization, and control. Bystanders do their best

M. Lynn
University of Miami Miller School of Medicine, Jackson Memorial Hospital,
Department of Surgery, Miami, FL, USA
e-mail: mlynn@med.miami.edu

© Springer Nature Switzerland AG 2019
M. Lynn et al. (eds.), *Disasters and Mass Casualty Incidents*,
https://doi.org/10.1007/978-3-319-97361-6_2

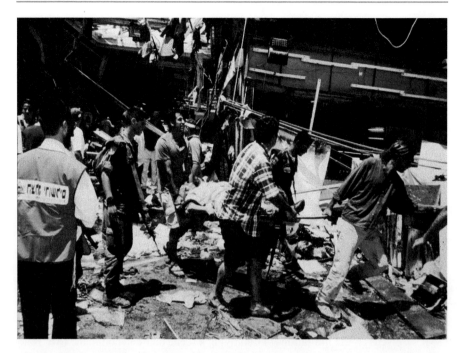

Fig. 2.1 Chaos phase after a market explosion in Jerusalem: Evacuation of injured patients performed by bystanders

to help, but their efforts are uncoordinated and at times can even exacerbate the already dangerous situation. The arrival of the first ambulances at the scene is not coordinated, and there is little control of their destination. It is during this phase that *minor injuries are evacuated first*, by private vehicles or by ambulances. As a result, these noncritical patients will be the first to arrive at local hospitals. Awareness of this phenomenon will ensure that the emergency rooms will not be filled and overwhelmed with minor injuries before the critical patients arrive.

It is almost impossible to control the chaos! The presence of "yellow tape" surrounding the scene does not mean the chaos, or the scene is under control!

Clearing the scene, by rapid evacuation of the critically injured, is a key strategy to reduce the chaos time. (Fig. 2.1).

Reorganization Phase

This is the second phase of a SMCI, and it starts when a scene incident command system (SIC) is activated, and the event is controlled. It is characterized by the presence of an incident commander (IC), who has the overall management responsibility for the event. During a SMCI, the IC is the first qualified person on scene. This could be a senior paramedic, a police officer, or a fire fighter. The IC remains in this position until this task is delegated to another authorized individual, and this

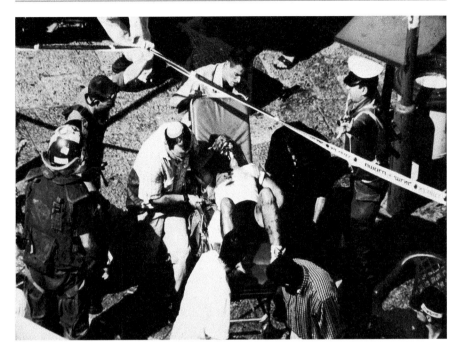

Fig. 2.2 Reorganization phase after a SMCI: EMS, fire, and police at the scene performing orderly evacuation of injured patients

transfer of command follows strict guidelines that includes a face-to-face meeting and a full debriefing.

It is during the reorganization phase that access and evacuation routes for ambulances are opened, proper triage of patients is performed, and the injured patients are distributed evenly among local hospitals, according to their medical needs. (Fig. 2.2).

Evacuation of Nonurgent Casualties

The final phase is the evacuation of the walking wounded, which typically comprises the vast majority of patients in a SMCI.

Note: With appropriate prehospital planning in combination with frequent live drills, all three phases of a SMCI should be completed within 60 to 90 min.

Incident Command System (ICS)

As mentioned previously, a sudden mass casualty incident (SMCI) is characterized by an event that occurs without prior notice. Therefore, the medical response to this type of incident should be seamless, well-coordinated, and immediate.

The deployment and setup of an incident command system (ICS) should be tailored in accordance to the magnitude of the event and the estimated time necessary for its conclusion. Not all incidents require a fully staffed and equipped ICS.

Incident Command Post (ICP) It is field location, at which the primary tactical-level and on-scene incident command functions are performed. The ICP may be located with the incident base or other incident command facilities and is normally identified by a green rotating or flashing light.

The Base of Operations (BoO) or Base in ICS terminology, is the location at which the primary logistics functions are coordinated and administered. The incident command post (ICP) may be co-located with the base. There is only one BoO per incident. The BoO is also where significant equipment maintenance, repair, reorder, and procurement activities occur. Finally, the BoO is where task force managers plan and coordinate the various interrelated functions, which enable the emergency operations to meet mission objectives as effectively and safely as possible.

A typical ICS should have the following components:
- Incident commander (IC).
- Command section (liaison officer, safety officer, and information officer): Responsible for developing, directing, and maintaining communications with multiple agencies on site. They work with local and public officials as well as media, to provide up to date information regarding the incident.
- Operations section (police, fire, medical): Responsible for handling tactical operations, coordinates the command objectives, and organizes all resources to the disaster site.
- Planning section: Provides the necessary information to the command center to develop the action plan. They also collect and evaluate information as it becomes available.
- Logistics section: Provides personnel equipment and support to the command center. They handle the coordination of all services involved in the response.
- Financial/administrative section: Responsible for accounting for funds that are used during the response and recovery aspect of the incident.

Sections are further broken down into units or branches. Branches can be further broken down into divisions and then into teams. (Fig. 2.3).

Examples
In an event of a mass shooting or an open-air explosion, injured patients will usually be visible and easily found. In such a situation, once the scene has been secured, the priority is to rapidly evacuate the critical victims to area hospitals. Delays in patient transport, with the sole purpose to set up a "formal" ICS, will negatively impact their outcome. In this type of event, an authoritative and

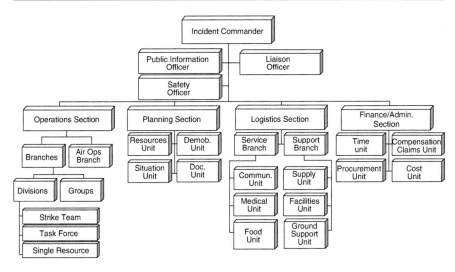

Fig. 2.3 Incident command structure – FEMA

well-trained paramedic, police officer or fire fighter should be sufficient to assume the role of incident commander and control the access and exit of fire trucks and ambulances, to and from the scene, and facilitate the even distribution of victims among local hospitals.

On the other hand, some events are more protracted such as train derailments, earthquakes, terrorist incidents or hostage situations, where victims maybe trapped inside the cars or collapsed buildings or when secondary explosive devices are suspected. These scenarios will require additional specialized resources such as

- Urban search and rescue (USAR).
- Hazardous material (HAZMAT teams).
- Explosive detection units (bomb squad) if scene safety is questionable.
- S.W.A.T. Units.

In these scenarios, establishing a formal ICS is vital (Fig. 2.4).

Adequate communications between all first responders working at the scene is imperative. In this type of event, the following items are the key duties of the IC and the ICS:

- Assure safety of the bystanders and the first responders.
- Assess the safety of the collapsed structure.
- Facilitate search and rescue.
- Provide command structure for S.W.A.T. Units.
- Provide open routes for patient transport.
- Communicate with the regional emergency operations center (REOC).
- Coordinate medically adequate distribution of patients to local hospitals (Fig. 2.5).

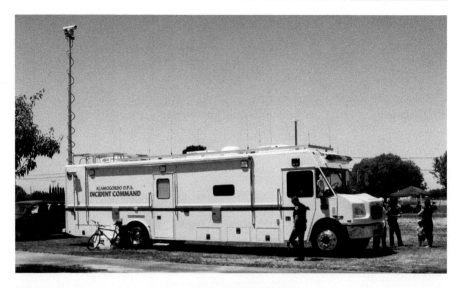

Fig. 2.4 A complete incident command vehicle ready to deploy.

Fig. 2.5 Incident command vehicle at the "Pulse" mass shooting to manage a hostage situation, Orlando, 2016

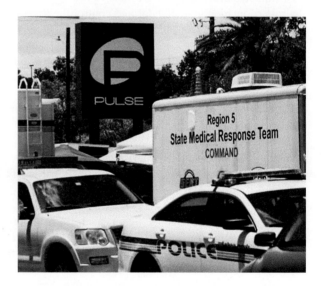

Regional Emergency Operations Center

Emergency Operations Center The emergency operations center (EOC) is the physical location where the coordination of information and resources to support domestic incident management activities normally takes place. An EOC may be at a temporary location or may be situated in a more central or permanently established facility. The structure of an EOC may comprise major functional disciplines (e.g., fire, law enforcement, and medical services), by jurisdiction (e.g., Federal, State, regional, county, city, tribal), or some combination thereof.

In principle, the main function of a regional emergency operations center (REOC), from a medical perspective, should be to shorten scene time of the first responders, by providing more assets such as ambulances and personnel when requested and coordinate the even distribution of patients among local hospitals.

In reality, the deployment of a fully staffed REOC is a time-consuming process, therefore, has limited value in SMCIs. In an event where search and rescue are not needed and rapid evacuation of victims to hospitals is the main priority, waiting to staff the REOC will certainly delay patient transport and negatively impact their outcome.

On the other hand, a fully operational REOC, incident command post and base of operations are of great value in sudden but protracted MCIs, where patients may be trapped in train cars or collapsed buildings, and even more so during progressive disasters such as biological epidemics, hurricanes, and planned mass gatherings. In these situations, a fully deployed and staffed REOC should be operational and have the following responsibilities (Fig. 2.6):

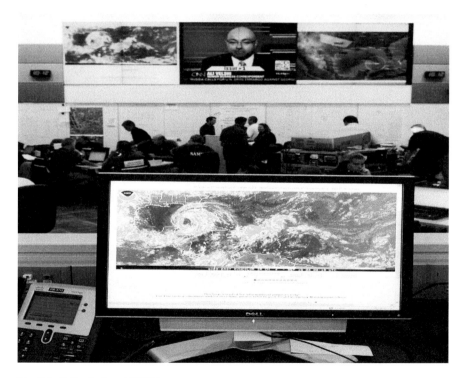

Fig. 2.6 Fully deployed REOC

- Assist with the search and rescue, providing personnel and equipment as requested by the incident commander (IC).
- Coordinate patient transport to the right hospital as dictated by his medical condition.
- Avoid overcrowding local hospitals by evenly distributing the patients.
- Estimate when local hospitals are overwhelmed and coordinated external assistance.
- Coordinate interhospital transfers, according to medical needs of the patients and bed availability.

Prehospital Communications

During normal operations, radio communication in the prehospital environment is confined within the respective agencies, with distinct frequencies for police department (PD), fire department (FD), and emergency medical services (EMS).

In a SMCI, there is a need for all first responders to communicate among themselves for better control and coordination at the scene. Nevertheless, in a large-scale SMCI such as Madrid train bombing and September 11, 2001, where hundreds of first responders were involved, one radio frequency for all would have been dysfunctional.

Another important issue is despite the need to have individualized response planning for progressive disasters and SMCIs, there cannot be distinct radio frequencies for each of those types of events.

Therefore, the communications plan for a progressive disaster or for a SMCI should include the following circles of communication and should be applied in accordance to the type of event, the speed of its progression, the deployment of an ICP and a REOC or at the discretion of the IC:

- Two police frequencies:
  - Between all police cars and the police officer staffing the ICP.
  - Between the police officer staffing the ICP and the police officer staffing the REOC.
- Two fire frequencies:
  - Between all fire trucks and the fire fighter staffing the ICP.
  - Between the fire fighter staffing the ICP and the fire fighter staffing the REOC.
- Two EMS frequencies:
  - Between all ambulances and the paramedic staffing the ICP.
  - Between the paramedic staffing the ICP and the paramedic staffing the REOC.
- One common emergency channel:
  - There should be one distinct frequency, to be used by all first responders during exceptional circumstances and at the discretion of the IC.
  - The emergency channel should be used during small-scale sudden events, when not many people are listening to this frequency or when an important

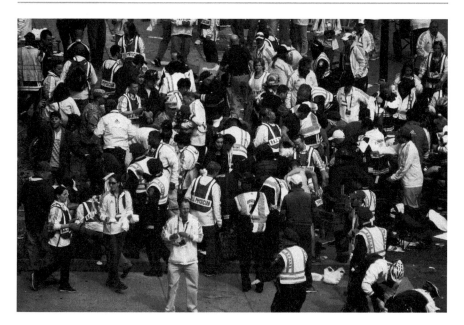

Fig. 2.7 The scene in the aftermath of the Boston Marathon Bombing and the importance of having a common emergency channel among all first responders

message needs to be transmitted immediately and is relevant to all first responders.
- The mechanism for all first responders to change from their specific frequency to the common emergency channel is to announce on their specific frequency that at a certain time (e.g., 10 a.m sharp), all vehicles need to change to the emergency frequency.

The communications plan should also include abbreviated communication codes to be spoken on the radio.

Important to stress that radio communication IS NOT a substitute for telephone and the importance of a strict radio discipline, as well as face-to-face communication. (Fig. 2.7).

Field Triage

As mentioned previously, the most clinically relevant definition of a SMCI is a *"temporary state of insufficiency."* From a prehospital perspective, it implies that in the first minutes after a SMCI, there may be the insufficient number of ambulances, personnel, equipment, limited access roads to the scene of the incident and few evacuation routes for the ambulances to transport the injured patients. Therefore, a simple and rapid triage needs to be performed to ensure that the critical patients are identified, managed and transported first. The SALT method of triage, SALT – sort assess life-saving interventions and treatment/transport, was developed as a national initial triage standard for all patients (e.g., adults, children, special populations).

S – sort patients into three groups, those who can move/walk to a designated area, those who can perform purposeful movements or wave and finally those who do not respond to verbal commands or are motionless.

A – assess begins with limited rapid assessment for life threatening injuries or conditions. The assessment should not take more than 1 min to perform.

L – life-saving interventions are simple. Critical interventions may be life saving and include
• Opening the airway with basic maneuvers.
• Hemorrhage control with direct pressure or a tourniquet.
• Insertion of a needle to the chest to relieve tension pneumothorax.

These interventions should take less than a few minutes, and they do not require the provider to remain with the patient for a prolonged period of time.

T – Transport: As patients receive their tags from the SALT process, they should move, as quickly as possible, to an ambulance for transport to a receiving facility.

Note: Moving patients to collection points/treatment area should occur only if ambulances are not available for transport.

The person that performs field triage (in different parts of the world, it could be a paramedic, EMT, or MD) needs to answer to three simple questions:
• *Who needs immediate care in the field?* (e.G., airway management).
• *Who needs immediate transport?* (e.G., internal hemorrhage that requires immediate surgical intervention).
• *Who can wait?* (e.G., mild injury or expectant).

Notes:
• Not all patients who require immediate airway management need necessarily to be transported first!
• The most important factor for the survival of a patient with internal hemorrhage is the speed to an operating room. Therefore, bleeding patients are the ones who should be transported first.
• The labeling the patients according to the severity of injury should be simple and fast, and should not delay transport to hospitals.
• The current acceptable triage categories are as follows:
    – Green: Minor injury – Walking wounded
    – Yellow: Delayed – Serious, not life threatening
    – Red: Immediate life-threatening injury
    – Black: Expectant/deceased (Fig. 2.8)
• During transport to the hospital, the condition of the patient may deteriorate. Therefore, it is important too perform additional triage upon arrival at the medical facility (Fig. 2.9).

Fig. 2.8 Example of triage tag used at field exercise

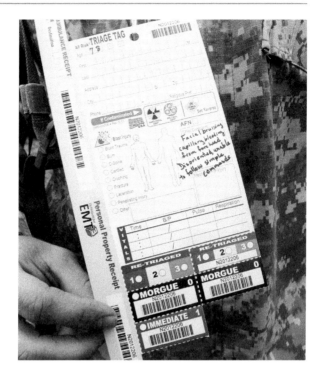

The Role of Bystanders and Volunteers in Sudden Mass Casualty Incidents

One of the most overlooked topics in disaster medicine is the role and the handling of bystanders following of a SMCI.

One would think that more assistance after an event, with multiple injured patients, would be beneficial. Nevertheless, it is conceivable that the presence of untrained individuals at the scene of a bombing, where secondary devices could be present, in the proximity of unstable buildings in the aftermath of an earthquake or inside contaminated areas after a radioactive or chemical spill, may add to the problem rather than help with the solution. In addition, medical management of injured patients by untrained persons may worsen their medical condition. A recent example was the Boston marathon bombing (Fig. 2.10). The application of improvised and inappropriately positioned tourniquets by bystanders appeared to have increased the bleeding from extremities of injured spectators.

In reality, however, it may be impossible to control the flow of bystanders during the chaos phase of a SMCI. However, once command and control are achieved (reorganization phase), the employment of bystanders, if necessary, should follow a few important guidelines:

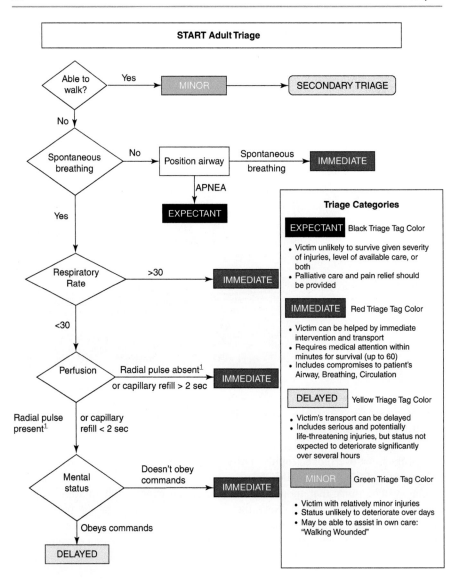

Fig. 2.9 The "START" adult triage system

What to do:

• Specific skills: It is common to find individuals with specific skills (doctors, nurses, paramedics, ex-military) within a large crowd of people. Utilization of these specific volunteers by the incident commander (IC) should be encouraged, providing that they fit into the incident command system (ICS). Medical personnel may provide assistance with the medical care and ex-military may be asked to assist with the evacuation of other spectators by controlling certain areas of the scene and managing other volunteers.

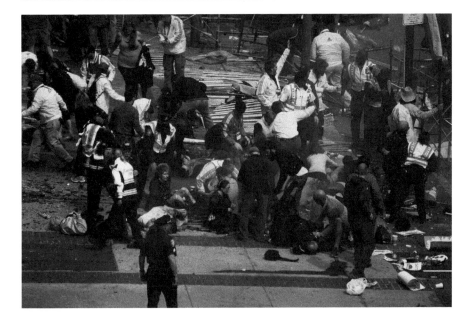

Fig. 2.10 Bystanders at the Boston Marathon Bombing

- Transporters: Volunteers may help by carrying stretchers to ambulances or may assist walking wounded patients to get to the closest place where medical attention could be provided.

What not to do:
- Safety: The most important objective is to assure the safety of the bystanders participating in the rescue efforts. If safety cannot be guaranteed, the employment of bystanders should be discouraged.
- Basic medical training: Volunteers should be allowed to manage injured patients only if they possess basic medical knowledge and training. When it comes to hemorrhage control, direct pressure on bleeding lacerations should be the only procedure performed by bystanders to control the bleeding. Persons *without any training* should not be allowed to place tourniquets or to use belts, cloths, and ropes as improvised tourniquets.
- Hospital staff deploying to the scene: Doctors and nurses should be discouraged to leave the hospitals to assist with the search and rescue efforts at the scene of the incident. It was one of the most important lessons learned from the Oklahoma City bombing.
- Urban search and rescue (USAR) is a profession that requires specific personnel with adequate knowledge and in-depth training. Furthermore, medical professionals with no experience of working in the field or in a hostile environment will quickly find themselves overwhelmed, unprepared, and they can easily become part of the problem.

"Save and Run" in Mass Casualty Incidents

The concept of *"Scoop and Run"* in trauma care originated to address those patients with massive internal bleeding and was employed successfully during the Korean War. It implies loading the patient to an ambulance, with minimal medical care at the scene, and transporting the patient, as quickly as possible, to an appropriate medical center, which can handle the injuries. In the US, it is usually a level I or II trauma center.

Yet, after conventional SMCIs, in addition to internal bleeding, patients may suffer other injuries, such as traumatic brain injury, tension pneumothorax, mangled extremities, or limb amputations.

In such situations, it becomes necessary to perform a few life-saving interventions prior to or during transport.

These interventions include:

- Airway management and ventilatory support.
- Needle thoracostomy for tension pneumothorax.
- Tourniquet placement for extremity bleeding.
- Note: If necessary, IV should be inserted only during transport and *should not* delay patient evacuation.

This is the concept of *"Save and Run,"* originally described by the Israeli EMS, implies performing these few life-saving procedures prior or during transport to hospitals (Fig. 2.11).

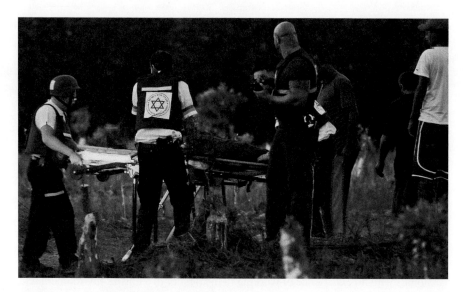

Fig. 2.11 Israeli EMS (MDA) at the scene

Distribution of Patients Between Hospitals and Prehospital Patient Tracking

There are a few important topics to consider when distributing patients between hospitals after a SMCI:
- Clinical diagnosis of the patient.
- Specific injuries: Traumatic brain injury (TBI), vascular, burns.
- Clinical capabilities of the hospitals in the area of the SMCI.
- Total number of injured to be evacuated.
- Number of critical patients.
- Number of ambulances available.
- Number of helicopters available.
- Distance of the local and regional hospitals to the incident.
- Avoidance of overwhelming hospitals.
- Use of "triage hospital" concept (details in the "hospital planning" section).

There are two types of methods for distribution of patients between hospitals:
- *Primary distribution:* The patient is transported to the definitive hospital, which has very specific capabilities and resources to adequately address the patients' injuries (Fig. 2.12).
- This is the preferred method and the best for the patient, since it allows for the shortest time to definitive care.

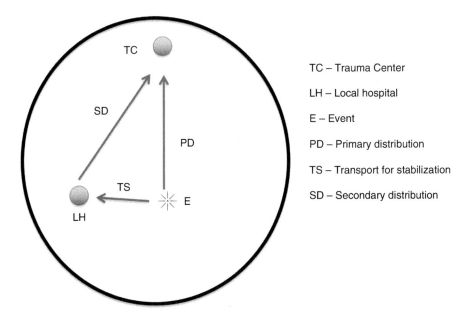

TC – Trauma Center

LH – Local hospital

E – Event

PD – Primary distribution

TS – Transport for stabilization

SD – Secondary distribution

Fig. 2.12 Primary vs. secondary distribution

- Nevertheless, if the distance to the definitive hospital is long and there are many casualties, it will require *many ambulances*, which may not be available, at least during the initial phase of a SMCI.
- The presence of *helicopters* may facilitate and expedite the transport of critical patients or specific types of injuries to definitive hospitals, while allowing ambulances to perform shorter transport times to local hospitals.
- *Secondary distribution:* Patient is transported to the nearest hospital ("triage hospital") and only after stabilization is the patient transferred to the definitive hospital (Fig. 2.12).
- With this method, ambulances will perform shorter transportation trips, thus, allowing for evacuation of a larger number of patients in a shorter period of time. However, this benefit will come at the cost of delaying definitive care for the patients with specific injuries.
- In addition, *secondary distribution* of patients requires a large number of ambulances and is associated with the huge logistical challenge of interhospital transport (Fig. 2.13). In this situation, the involvement of the regional emergency operations center (REOC) is imperative.
- Note:
- In a large-scale *urban SMCI*, where trauma centers may be close to the event, it is possible to use large helicopters (military) to distribute the mildly injured patients (which account for the vast majority) to distant hospitals rather than to the trauma centers in the area. This concept has two benefits:
  - Will allow the trauma centers to focus their efforts on the critically injured.
  - Reduce the risks of air transport of critically injured patients.

The decision about the preferred method of patient distribution is the responsibility of the incident commander in coordination with the REOC, with the above considerations.

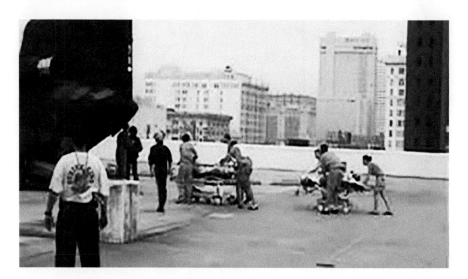

Fig. 2.13 Hospital patient evacuation during Katrina

Prehospital Patient Tracking

Large-scale urban SMCIs are overwhelming events to any city. The initial chaos phase may be longer than expected. Control and coordination between ambulances may be lacking. As a result, change in ambulance destination after leaving the scene is typical.

Thus, the use of prehospital patient-tracking devices, such as barcode scanners (Fig. 2.14), will not only delay patient evacuation but may also be inaccurate, causing confusion to incident managers and families.

Tracking of patients is important but should be used, almost exclusively, at the hospitals.

Difference Between Urban and Rural Sudden Mass Casualty Incidents

Urban (Fig. 2.15):
• Trauma centers immediately available within close proximity.
• Larger number of ambulances readily available.
• Scarce use of air transport.
• Most common method of patient distribution: Primary.

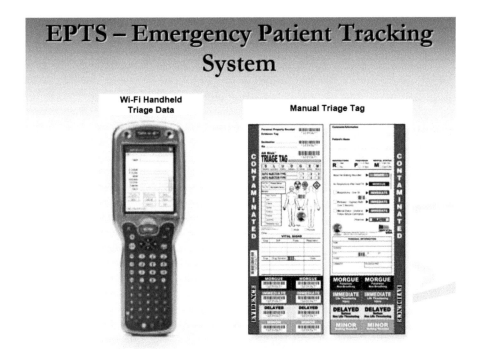

Fig. 2.14 Prehospital tracking of patients

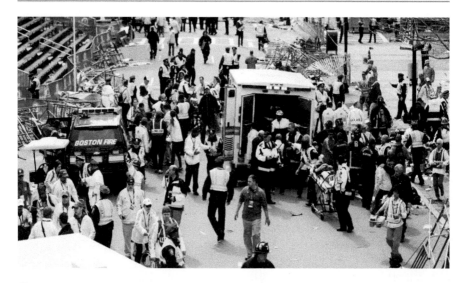

Fig. 2.15 Boston Marathon Bombing, 2013

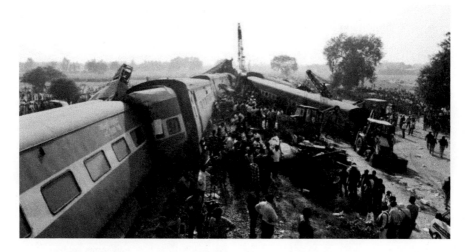

Fig. 2.16 Train derailment in rural area, India, 2016

Rural (Fig. 2.16):
- Longer time to definitive care and to trauma centers.
- Fewer ambulances available, requires mobilization of ambulances and resources from other counties.
- Air transport is usually needed for critical patients.
- Most common method of patient distribution: Secondary.
- The use of the "triage hospital" concept is common.

Hospital Planning and Response to Sudden Mass Casualty Incidents

3

Mauricio Lynn

Introduction

This chapter describes the essential topics that a hospital needs to address when planning the response to a sudden mass casualty incident (SMCI). It describes in detail the major components of a hospital plan, how to acutely increase hospital capacity and plan alternate treatment areas, how to quickly activate the plan, the challenges with identification and registration of multiple patients simultaneously, and finally how to handle large numbers of families, friends, and media.

Essentials Components of a Sudden Mass Casualty Incident Plan

Introduction

The differences between progressive disasters and SMCI's were addressed previously.

From a medical perspective, there are many clinical, logistical, and organizational differences between the various types of progressive disasters and SMCIs; therefore, planning should specific for each type.

Written plans should be detailed and specific for:
- Conventional/burn MCIs
- Chemical/toxicological MCIs
- Radiation incidents
- Biological disasters

M. Lynn
University of Miami Miller School of Medicine, Jackson Memorial Hospital,
Department of Surgery, Miami, FL, USA
e-mail: mlynn@med.miami.edu

© Springer Nature Switzerland AG 2019
M. Lynn et al. (eds.), *Disasters and Mass Casualty Incidents*,
https://doi.org/10.1007/978-3-319-97361-6_3

The hospital plan should be the same for weekdays, weeknights, weekends, and holidays.

A hospital plan for a SMCI should include the following components:

- Strategies to prevent patients flooding the hospital
- Surge capacity specific for the hospital: The resources (staff, space, supplies) needed to manage a sudden surge in the number of patients, above its normal capacity (see next chapter)
- Method for call-in of additional personnel
- Organization of treatment areas
- Opening and organization of alternate treatment sites
- Deployment of additional equipment and supplies to existing and alternate treatment sites
- Hospital communications plan
- Method of Identification of patients, registration, and patient tracking
- Individualized plan for respiratory therapy, blood bank, laboratory, radiology
- Organization of a family/friends information center
- Activation of the SMCI plan and hospital response
- Triage and principles of medical care during a SMCI
- Planning and activation of hospital decontamination for chemical exposure

Hospital Surge Capacity Calculation

Assumptions and Definitions

Hospital planning for SMCIs and disasters assumes that the hospital is at full capacity, including the emergency department and the intensive care unit(s).

Hospital surge capacity (HSC) is the acute augmentation of its capacity, to receive and manage victims of a SMCI.

The components of HSC are additional *staff*, alternate *space*, and extra *equipment and supplies* (Fig. 3.1).

Note *Absence of empty beds in the ED or at the hospital is not a requirement for acute surge capacity panning. There is not one ED in the world that has 10–20 open beds waiting for a SMCI to occur!*

The importance of computing HSC specific to each medical center is to have an estimate of the maximal number of additional patients to be treated at the institution and consequently the number of additional personnel, critical equipment, supplies, and stretchers (that will be used as additional beds) that need to be deployed after a SMCI.

Obviously, a 500-bed hospital will have a different HSC than a 1000-bed hospital.

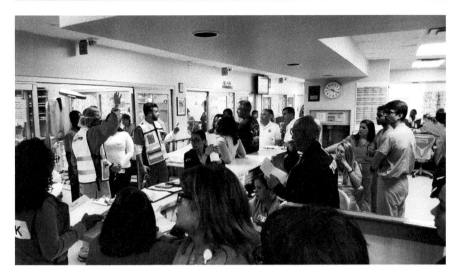

Fig. 3.1 Debriefing of staff during a SMCI drill, Ryder Trauma Center, Miami, 2018

Maximal Number of Patients (MNP) Per Hospital

The maximal number of additional patients to be treated at any given hospital during a SMCI is approximately 20% of the total bed capacity of the hospital.

Example *Hospital with 500 licensed beds will manage up to 100 casualties.*

Of the MNP, up to 20% of all victims will be pediatric patients.

Of the MNP, up to 30% of patients will have different degrees of posttraumatic stress disorder (PTSD), distinct or in conjunction with conventional injuries.

Distribution of Victims by Severity

For planning purposes, it is assumed that the *maximum number of critical patients* that could be treated at any hospital will not exceed 20% of MNP. This number has important implications in terms of additional personnel, critical equipment (such as ventilators), and number of extra stretchers (used as temporary extra beds) needed to manage the sudden surge of patients.

Table 3.1 below summarizes the distribution of patients, by severity, to be treated at any medical facility after a SMCI:

Example *A 500-bed hospital will manage up to 20 critical patients.*

A hospital plan for a SMCI needs to identify areas in the emergency department or other alternate sites, to concentrate patients by severity. A physician-in-charge needs to be appointed to each site.

Table 3.1 Distribution of injuries by severity

Severity	% of MNP
Reds – Severe (Life threatening)	20
Yellow – Moderate (Limb/eye threatening)	30
Green – Mild, walking wounded	50

Table 3.2 Personnel planning for ED intake, initial evaluation, and management

Personnel/staff	Triage	Severe	Moderate	Mild	Mental	Pediatrics
Attending/fellow[a]	1	1	1	1	1	1
Physician/patient ratio (MD)		1/1	1/10	1/10	1/3	1/10
Nurse/patient ratio (RN)	2 RN	1/1	1/5	1/5	1/3	1/5
Respiratory therapist (RT)	n/a	1/4	n/a	n/a	n/a	n/a
Escort/patient ratio (ES)	1/10	1/3	1/10	1/10	1/10	1/10
Clerk/patient ratio (CL)	1–2 CL	1/2	1/5	1/5	1/5	1/5
Radiology technicians (RD)	n/a	1/5	1/10	1/10	n/a	1/10
Blood bank runners (BB)	n/1	1/10	1/20	n/a	n/a	n/a
Security guards (SG)	5–10	1	1	1	1	1
Administrator[b] (AD)	1	1	1	1	1	1

[a]Attending/fellow relates to teaching hospitals
[b]Assists the physician-in-charge/charge nurse with administration and logistics
n/a not applicable

Table 3.2 below summarizes the number of personnel required to manage patients from a SMCI, according to severity. A hospital is required to have an emergency call-in list to bring back critical personnel if a SMCI occurs after hours, on weekends or holidays.

Example *In the first hour, a hospital with 500 licensed beds will need to have available about:*
- *20 doctors.*
- *20 nurses.*
- *Five respiratory therapists.*
- *10 escorts.*
- *10 clerks.*
- *Five radiology technicians.*
- *Two blood bank technicians.*
- *10 security guards.*
- *Three administrators.*

The purpose of the above personnel is to triage, transport, register, evaluate, and manage the initial flow of patients. The priority is to manage the severe/critical patients first!
About *10% of the severe casualties* from a conventional SMCI will require emergent life-saving surgery. About half of those will require hemorrhage control, while the other half will require neurosurgical interventions.

Table 3.3 Approximate number of urgent operations, as function of the MNP

Operation	% of MNP
Open fractures	10
Penetrating eye injuries	5
Neurological (urgent)	10
Chest	5
Oral/maxillary/facial	5–10
Burns	5–10

Table 3.4 Critical equipment/supplies planning

Equipment	% of MNP
Stretchers	35 (% of Reds + ½ of Yellows)
Wheelchairs	65 (% of Greens + ½ of yellows)
Ventilators	20 (% of Reds)
Cardiac monitors	35 (% of Reds + ½ Yellows)
Pulse oxymeters	20 (% of Reds)
Trauma carts (each cart for 20 patients)	# of carts = MNP-ED capacity/20
ICU carts (each cart for 20 patients)	# of carts = # of reds/20

Example *A 500-bed hospital will manage up to 20 severe/critical patients of which about 2 will need emergency life-saving surgery (10% of 20). Therefore, this hospital will need to have available two immediate operating rooms, one to two general/ trauma surgery teams, and one neurosurgical team.*

A significant number of patients will require one or more surgical interventions during their hospital stay. These procedures are considered urgent.

Table 3.3 below shows the approximate percentage of victims who will require urgent surgery by specialty:

Table 3.4 summarizes the total amount of critical equipment and supplies necessary, as function of the MNP, to manage a SMCI at a 500-bed hospital.

Treatment Areas, Alternate Sites, and Deployment of Extra Equipment and Supplies

Principles

- In a SMCI, there may be insufficient space to manage the abrupt surge of patients.
- It is important to concentrate patients, according to severity, in *one* area.
- In addition to the treatment areas in the emergency department (ED) or trauma center (TC – if applicable), there is a need to designate alternate treatment areas to cope with the sudden increase of patients.
- The number of alternate treatment areas will be in accordance to the calculated maximal number of patients (MNP) specific for the hospital, as discussed previously.

Designated Treatment Areas

- Severe/critical patients (Reds):
  - ED
  - Trauma center (if applicable) (Fig. 3.1)
- Urgent patients (Yellows):
  - ED
  - Alternate site
- Mild injuries (Greens):
  - Alternate site (hospital lobby, ambulatory care center)
- Pediatric patients:
  - Pediatric ED (if applicable)
  - Alternate site
- Mental health:
  - Ambulatory care center
  - Alternate
- Alternate intensive care unit (ICU):
  - Operating room recovery

Sources of Personnel for the Treatment Areas

- Regular ED and/or TC personnel
- Call-in personnel
- ICU nurses from ICU(s)
- See hospital surge capacity estimation for the number of personnel required, as function of severity

Equipment and Supplies

- Stretchers will serve as extra beds at the alternate treatment sites.
- Trauma carts: Each cart stocked with supplies for 20 patients.
- ICU carts: Each cart stocked with supplies for 20 patients.
- Extra ventilators.
- Communications (as per hospital communication plan for SMCIs) (Fig. 3.2).

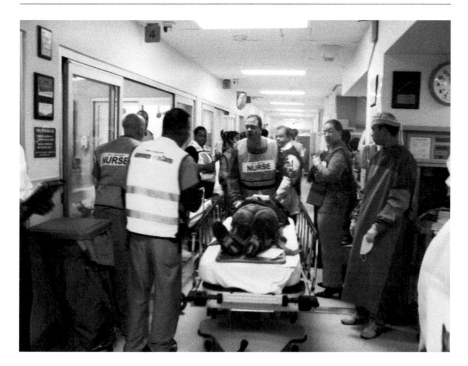

Fig. 3.2 "Red" patients transported to Ryder Trauma Center during MCI drill, Miami, 2018

Hospital Communications During Sudden Mass Casualty Incidents

Assumptions

During a SMCI, there is a need to have flow of information to and from the hospital and within the hospital simultaneously.

Landlines may be affected during flooding and overwhelmed during a SMCI; therefore, there is a need for other means of communication.

Utilization of personal cell phones may be an option. Nevertheless, depending on the carrier, signal strength may vary within the hospital. In addition, cellular towers may be affected during earthquakes.

Therefore, handheld professional *two-way radios* may be an excellent alternative (Fig. 3.1).

Channels (Frequencies)

At least two communications channels should be available at the hospital:
- Security channel
- Medical channel
- It is important to have a distinct medical channel to communicate between the important areas of the hospital respective to patient care and logistics.
    - Triage area
    - Treatment sites in emergency department (ED) and trauma center (TC)
    - Operating room
    - Respiratory therapy
    - Transport
    - Blood bank
    - Radiology
    - Laboratory
    - Security
    - Incident command center
    - Family/friends information center

Below is a suggested list of functions that need to be on the medical frequency:
- Hospital disaster manager/representative
- Surgeon in charge of the event (for conventional SMCI)
- Radiology supervisor
- Respiratory supervisor
- Clerk supervisor
- Patient staging supervisor
- Triage officer
- ED physician-in-charge
- ED charge nurse
- Pediatric ED physician-in-charge (where applicable)
- Pediatric ED charge nurse (where applicable)
- Physician-in-charge of the RED treatment area
- Physician-in-charge of the YELLOW treatment area
- Physician-in-charge of the GREEN treatment area
- "Operating room priority" surgeon
- Senior anesthesiologist on call
- Blood bank
- Transport supervisor
- Social services/family information center
- Trauma center head/charge nurse (where applicable)
- Incident command center
- Supervisor at personnel meeting point (physicians and nurses) (Fig. 3.3)

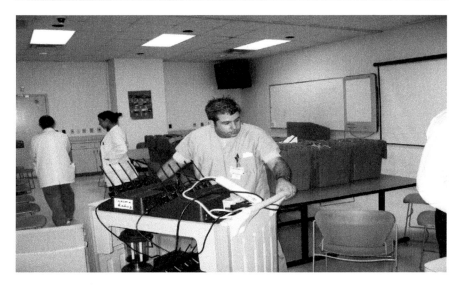

Fig. 3.3   Portable radios being distributed during a MCI drill, Ryder Trauma Center, Miami

The communications plan should also include abbreviated communication codes to be spoken on the radio.

Important to state that radio communication *IS NOT* a substitute for telephone or face-to-face communications and the importance of a strict radio discipline.

Activation of a Mass Casualty Plan

Activation

In principle, the activation of a SMCI plan must be simple and systematic, based on preprepared checklists.
- Notification:
- The notification that a possible SMCI has occurred will be to the emergency department (ED) or trauma center (TC) through one of the following ways:
  - Fire rescue radio
  - Direct land phone lines to the ED/TC
  - Through hospital operator
  - News media
  - First casualty or person arriving to the ED from the scene
  - From hospital security

Once the notification is received in the ED/TC, a brief discussion among the senior surgeon on call, the ED senior physician, and the ED/TC charge nurse(s) should occur to assess the situation and decide whether to activate the MCI plan.

- Verification:
  - Verify if the event is real – call back the regional emergency operations center (REOC)/ EMS, Police
  - Verify type of event: conventional/chemical/radiological ("dirty bomb")
  - Discuss event with ED physician/surgeon in charge and ED/TC charge nurse
- Approval to activate MCI plan:
- The formal activation of the MCI plan requires approval of the chief executive officer (CEO) of the hospital or his designee.
  - Call CEO/COO/CMO/CNO/executive on call to approve activation of SMCI plan.
  - Once activation of the MCI plan is approved, the senior surgeon, ED senior physician, and the ED/TC charge nurse will simultaneously complete their respective checklists, assuring maximal coordination.
- Senior surgeon/ED physician in charge checklist:
  - Activate in-house and call-in lists (if necessary, as function of magnitude of the event).
  - Get a portable radio.
  - Verify with ED/TC charge nurse creation of spaces in ED and alternate care sites.
  - Notify the operating room (OR) and cancel scheduled, nonurgent operations.
  - Verify that security, respiratory therapy, blood bank, radiology, laboratory, and mental health were notified.
  - Activate triage site: designates appropriate triage physician (surgeon/ED physician) according to availability.
  - Debrief arriving personnel about the event and briefly describe the management strategy.
  - Designate medical teams: 1MD, 1RN per patient for critical/severe (Red) patients.
  - Designate OR teams, as calculated by hospital size: (OR team = 1 surgeon or neurosurgeon, 1 surgical or neurosurgery assistant, one anesthesiologist, one anesthesia assistant, two OR nurses).
  - Designate "OR priority surgeon" (does not scrub). Once "OR priority surgeon" arrives, he/she takes charge of designating OR teams and prioritizing emergency operations.
  - Distribute call-in physicians, together with ED charge nurse, to form medical teams with nurses.
  - Designate administrative assistant to follow you (to hold your radio, update you about number of casualties, including age and severity).
  - Communicate frequently and update the hospital incident command center (phone/radio).
  - Perform frequent debriefings to the entire workforce about the magnitude of event and changes in management strategies (if applicable). Dismiss unnecessary personnel.

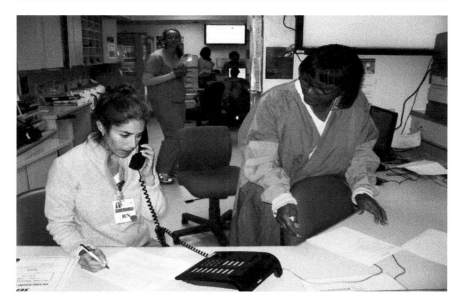

Fig. 3.4 Charge nurse activating disaster plan following checklist, Ryder Trauma Center, Miami

- ED Head/Charge nurse checklist (Fig. 3.4):
  - Notify security
  - Activate overhead paging system (if available)
  - Activate call-in lists (if necessary, as function of magnitude of the event)
    - Activate the disaster paging system/mass communication
  - Call ICU nurses to meeting point
  - Call all doctors in house to meeting point
  - Activate of the emergency stretchers plan. 20 stretchers and 20 wheelchairs immediately to triage area.
  - Empty ED (ventilated patients are not moved to alternate sites)
  - Notify and verify creation of spaces in alternate care sites
  - Notify OR
  - Notify blood bank (phone/radio), radiology (phone/radio), laboratory (phone/radio), mental health (phone/radio)
  - Activate emergency equipment plan:
    - Move additional ventilators to "ventilator concentration point"
    - Move trauma carts to ED/alternate care sites
    - Move ICU carts to preplanned alternate ICU site
  - Debrief arriving nurses about event and management plan
  - Distribute identification vests and radio communications
  - Form medical teams for arriving victims: 1 MD, 1 RN per critical/severe (Red) patient (team 1 – first arriving patient, team 2 – second arriving patient, etc.)
  - Distribute call-in arrivals (MDs and nurses arriving from home)

Call-In of Essential Personnel in a Sudden Mass Casualty Incident

The most important asset of hospital surge capacity is the ability to match the abrupt surge of patients during a SMCI with the adequate amount of essential personnel:
- Doctors
- Nurses
- Respiratory therapists
- Radiology technicians
- Laboratory technicians
- Blood bank technicians
- Clerks
- Transporters
- Security guards

During progressive disasters, approaching hurricanes, and planned sporting events, there is time to increase the amount of personnel needed to respond to a potential increase in the number of patients.

Nevertheless, in a SMCI, where the surge of patients is abrupt and without prior notice, acutely increasing the amount of personnel may be a true challenge. Therefore, a hospital needs to have redundant methods to rapidly and efficiently call-in personnel, once the hospital's SMCI plan is activated.

The source of additional personnel may be from
- Within the hospital
- From home

Methods for Call-In of Personnel

- Overhead paging system for the entire hospital
- Alphanumeric paging system
- Web-based "mass communicator" system

Note "Call-in tree" (Fig. 3.5): This method assumes the listed people are in town and will answer their phone. While adequate for progressive disasters, it should not be used as the main call-in process in SMCIs.

Identification Badges

- All personnel called from home need to have their identification badges at all time, to facilitate driving through police checkpoints.

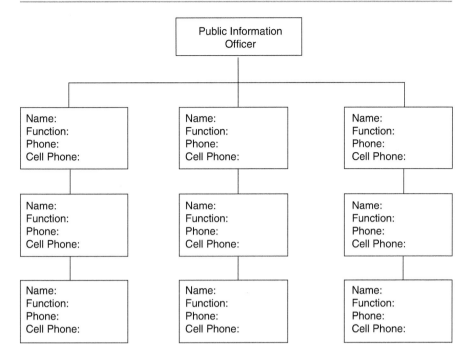

Fig. 3.5 Phone call-in tree

Parking

- The call-in plan should include a predesignated parking area in an event that there is need for extra parking space for the personnel arriving from home.

Meeting Points

- The call-in plan should include a designated meeting point for call-in of personnel. Its location should be in accordance to the specific function:
  - Clinical personnel should meet close to the treatment sites.
  - Respiratory therapists should meet where the ventilators are stored.
  - Radiology technicians should meet where the portable X-ray machines are stored.
  - Blood bank and laboratory technicians should meet at the laboratory.
  - Transporters/escorts should meet where the extra stretchers/wheel chairs are stored.
  - Registration clerks should meet at the administration offices.

Hospital Strategies to Prevent "Flooding" of Patients

It is possible that after a SMCI or a sudden chemical mass casualty incident (SCMCI), a large number of self-evacuated or mildly contaminated patients that are frightened and panicked, may attempt to burst into the hospital, despite all security measures.

After the Tokyo subway attack with sarin gas in 1995, 82% of contaminated casualties arrived at the hospitals driven by private cars, with consequent contamination of 25% of the hospital staff.

A large number of patients self-evacuated and transported to medical centers by bystanders after the mass shooting at the "Pulse" nightclub in Orlando (Fig. 3.6) and at the concert in Las Vegas.

Medical centers need to have the means to prevent uncoordinated flooding of patients and control their access to designated hospital triage areas.

Potential solutions:

- Security guards: It is highly unlikely that security guards will be able to contain dozens, if not hundreds of panicked individuals attempting to enter the hospital.
- Perimeter fence: A physical barrier, surrounding the entire medical center, is probably the best solution to control access of patients to the hospital.
- The perimeter fence should have gates (Fig. 3.7), which would remain open during normal hospital operation and can be quickly closed when the threat for a sudden overflow of patients exists, allowing access control of patients, families, and friends.

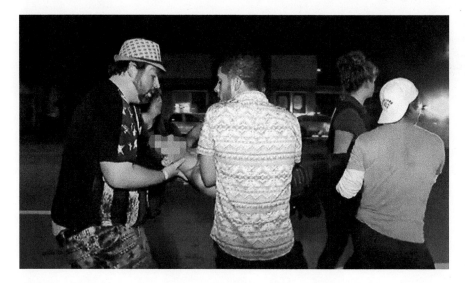

Fig. 3.6 Self-evacuation from the "Pulse" nightclub, Orlando, FL, 2016

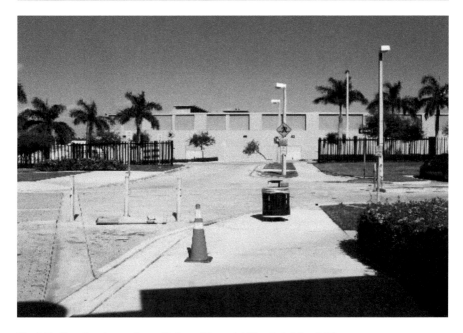

Fig. 3.7 Gated perimeter fence, Jackson Memorial Hospital, Miami, FL

Fig. 3.8 Exercise to
familiarize security guards
with gates closure
procedures

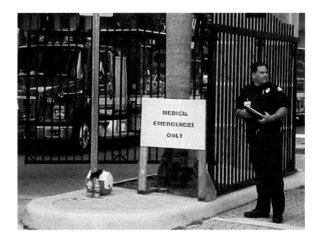

- The closure of the gates should be the responsibility of the Chief of Security of the hospital. After construction of the fence is completed, it is recommended to perform a few drills to familiarize the security guards with the procedures required to close the gates after the notification that a SMCI has occurred (Fig. 3.8).

Hospital Response: Preparation Triage Area and Emergency Department

Immediately after approval to activate the SMCI plan is received, as described previously, the hospital initiates its response to the incident.

The first priority is to prepare the triage area outside the emergency department (ED) and create space inside the ED for the incoming critical patients. Preferably, these processes should be performed simultaneously.

Preparation of "Stretchers Concentration Point"

- Transport (escort) supervisor will distribute transporters (escorts) to the triage area and ED and perform the following actions:
  - Deploy escorts to help create spaces in the ED.
  - Deploy escorts to open the stretchers storage (Fig. 3.9) and distribute the stretchers to the "stretcher concentration point," in proximity to the triage area and outside the ED (Fig. 3.10).
  - Escorts will bring all empty stretchers/wheelchairs from ED to the "stretcher concentration point" in proximity to the triage area and outside the ED (Figs. 3.11 and 3.12).
  - At the "stretcher concentration point," the escort supervisor will have radio communications, *on medical frequency*, with all treatment areas. He/she will deploy escorts according to demand.
  - A voice amplification device should be used to facilitate control of the area.

Fig. 3.9 Stretchers and wheelchairs storage located next to triage area

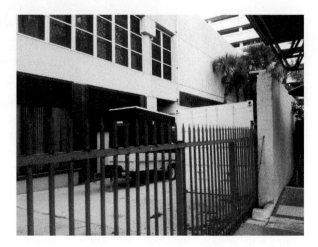

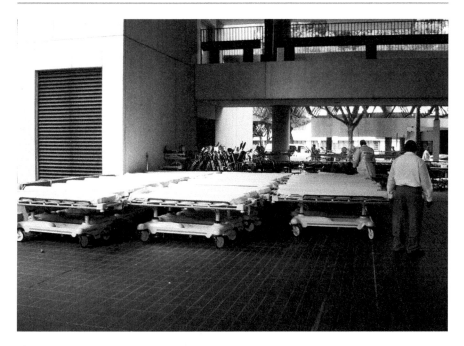

Fig. 3.10 "Stretcher concentration point" located next to the triage area

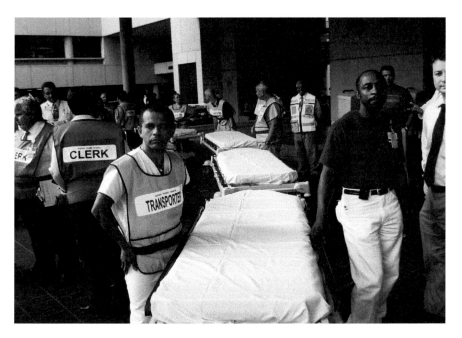

Fig. 3.11 Escorts at the "stretchers concentration point"

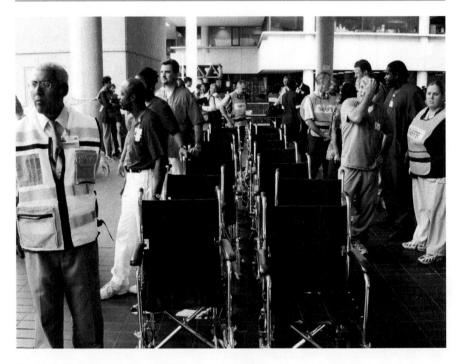

Fig. 3.12 Escorts at the "stretchers concentration point"

Preparation of Triage Area

- Personnel (Fig. 3.13):
    - Triage officer: Surgeon/ED physician/nurse practitioner
    - Two registered nurses from ED
    - Three or more clerks for quick patient registration, photography, and severity labeling according to the triage officer
- Equipment/supplies (Fig. 3.5):
    - Colored charts and arm bands: The total number of charts and arm bands will be determined according to the total number of patients expected to be managed at the institution.
    - The number of "Red," "Yellow," and "Green" charts and arm bands are according to the expected number of patients and their severity.
    - The charts and armbands should have predetermined registration numbers.
    - The charts should include basic documentation forms: rapid medical assessment, X-ray, and blood bank.
    - No documentation will be performed at triage area. *Only* categorization of severity.
    - Digital cameras should be used by one of the registration clerks to photograph comatose patients or infants. The temporary medical record number (T number) should be included in the picture.

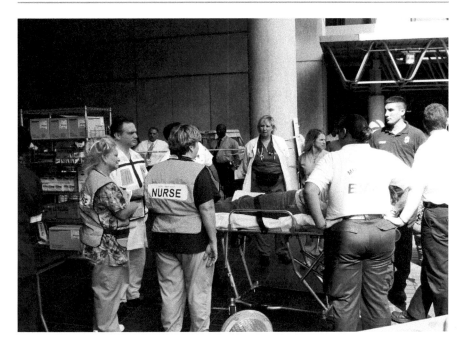

Fig. 3.13   Personnel and supplies at the triage area

- A voice amplification device should be used by the triage officer to facilitate control of the area.
- ED administrator, in consultation with ED charge nurse, is responsible for ensuring that these supplies are ready and available.

Evacuation of ED

- Simultaneously, the surgeon in charge and the ED physician will make decisions with regard to those patients who can be safely moved to other treatment areas.
  - Ventilated patients in the ED will be transferred out only if an ICU bed is available.
  - Patients from the ED area will be moved to available beds in the hospital. If no beds are available, patients will be placed in corridors, under nursing/medical supervision as needed.
  - Medically stable patients in the ED, identified by a physician and charge nurse, will be transported to preplanned alternate care areas. This space will serve as a staging area until floor beds are available. All patients will remain under nursing/medical supervision at all times.
  - ED surge capacity is based on availability of extra medical staff and space for the incoming patients, which will be transported to the ED on stretchers or wheelchairs from the triage area.

Preparation of ED and In-Hospital Treatment Sites

- Severe casualties site ("Red"):
  - All severe casualties will be treated in the trauma center (TC) (where applicable) or designated areas in the ED. In case there is a need for more space for severe casualties, patients will then be treated at alternate treatment sites, such as the recovery room of the operating room or another preplanned location.
  - The surgeon in charge of the severe casualties site is the surgeon on call. Other surgeons/doctors will be assigned to the site as they arrive and become available.
  - Nurses will be assigned to the site as they arrive from other hospital areas or from home.
  - Communications: Radio on medical frequency for surgeon and nurse in charge of the site.
  - Equipment: The standard equipment and supplies for trauma care already present in the ED will be used and supplemented by "trauma carts" as needed.
- Delayed casualties site ("Yellow"):
  - Delayed casualties will be treated at designated areas in the ED.
  - The surgeon in charge of delayed casualties site is a surgeon assigned by the surgeon in charge of the event. Other surgeons/doctors will be assigned to the site as they arrive and become available.
  - Nurses will be assigned to the site as they arrive from other hospital areas or from home.
  - Communications: Radio on Medical frequency for surgeon and nurse in charge of the site.
  - Equipment: The standard equipment and supplies for trauma care already present in the ED will be used and supplemented by "trauma carts" as needed.
- Mild casualties (walking-wounded) site ("Green"):
  - Mild casualties "Green" (the majority of the victims) will be treated at ambulatory care centers or other preplanned areas of the hospital. Walking wounded patients should NOT be allowed in the ED, until a complete assessment of the scene of the event is performed.
  - Usually, there is no need for stretchers for these patients; they can sit in a chair or wheel chair and wait for their turn to be examined.
  - The surgeon in charge of walking-wounded site is a surgeon assigned by the surgeon in charge of the event. Other surgeons/doctors will be assigned to the site as they arrive and become available.
  - Nurses will be assigned to the site as they arrive from other hospital areas or from home.
  - Communications: Radio on medical frequency for surgeon in charge and nurse in charge of the site.
  - Equipment: "Trauma carts" to be distributed as needed.
- Pediatric victims:
  - Pediatric casualties of conventional SMCI will be treated in the trauma center (where applicable) or the pediatric ED (where applicable) or the ED according to severity of injuries.

- The pediatric surgeon in charge of the event is the pediatric surgeon on call (where applicable). Other pediatric surgeons/doctors will be assigned as they arrive and become available.
- Nurses will be assigned to the site as they arrive from other hospital areas or from home.
- Communications: Radio on medical frequency for pediatric surgeon and nurse in charge of the site.
- Equipment: The standard equipment and supplies for trauma care already present in the Pediatric ED/ ED will be used and supplemented by "trauma carts" as needed.
- Mental health triage (MHT):
- Casualties demonstrating signs and symptoms of behavioral health concerns will be treated at the preplanned site for mental health patients.
  - The physician in charge of MHT is the psychiatrist/psychologist on call (where applicable).
  - Specific equipment, supplies, and drugs for mental health patients will be distributed as needed.
- Operating room:
  - The first patient who requires resuscitative surgery will be transferred to the OR, assuring that there is adequate staffing.
  - The surgeon in charge in the OR is one of the surgeons called in from home. His/her function is to be the "OR priority" surgeon. He/she will not scrub, unless it is absolutely necessary. His/her function is to prioritize patients to the OR, among the various requests from different services.
  - Emergency surgery priorities:
    - Life threatening:
      - Hemodynamic instability
      - Intracranial hematoma
    - Limb/organ threatening:
      - Vascular injury
      - Penetrating eye injury
    - Other priorities:
      - Peritonitis
      - Open fractures
      - Debridement of infected wounds/amputations (Fig. 3.14)
      - Excision of burns
  - Communications: Radio on medical frequency for "OR priority surgeon" and OR charge nurse. Intercom and telephones to be used as need and where applicable.
  - Personnel: It is the responsibility of OR supervisor/charge nurse to have OR staff for the calculated resuscitative operations within 30 min from event announcement.
  - Supplies: It is the responsibility of OR supervisor/charge nurse to have surgical supplies immediately available for the calculated resuscitative operations and adequate sterilization capabilities.

Fig. 3.14 Blast
amputation of left upper
extremity

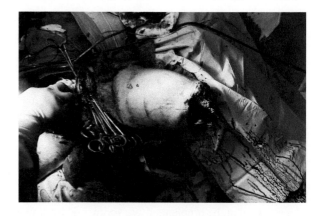

- Intensive care units:
  - Patients who require ICU beds will be admitted according to bed availability.
  - Alternate ICU beds need to be available according to SMCI plan.
  - Personnel: Available nurses from other intensive care units need to be redistributed by the hospital head nurse/designee, until arrival of ICU nurses called in from home.
  - Equipment and supplies: Ventilators and ICU carts at alternate sites to be distributed as needed.
- Respiratory therapy:
  - Immediately after event announcement, the respiratory supervisor in house should deliver five ventilators to the "ventilator concentration point," usually located in proximity to the ED/TC.
  - Other ventilators will be distributed to the treatment sites as needed.
  - Communications: Radio on medical frequency for the respiratory supervisor.
- Registration:
  - The clerk supervisor should deploy all clerks available in the hospital to the treatment sites as soon as possible after the activation of the MCI plan.
  - Communication: Radio on medical frequency for the clerk supervisor.

Hospital Response: Identification, Registration, Triage, and Inflow of Patients

The early stages of a SMCI are characterized by confusion and lack of command and control. It is called the "chaos" phase.

It is not uncommon for patients to be misidentified.

It is critical that a hospital have a mature identification and registration system, for multiple simultaneous patients and that could be easily accessed when tracking of patients is required by family members or friends looking for their loved ones.

Identification

Identification of comatose patients and/or infants should start at the triage area of the hospital. For this purpose, cameras should be used to photograph the face of the arriving patient together with the T-number associated with the appropriate colored chart. The pictures should be stored in a specific digital folder connected to the hospital information system (HIS) of the hospital. Pictures of unidentified patients are then shown to family members at the family/friends information center (FIC), discussed later in this section.

Registration

Simultaneous registration of multiple patients during a SMCI is a real challenge and of critical importance. It is common to misidentify comatose patients or infants that were close to other victims or may have been in possession of bags or wallets of their friends when the event occurred.

When planning for a SMCI, it is important to plan for enough clerks to register multiple injured simultaneously during the influx of patients. Calculation of the approximate number of clerks required for a given hospital was discussed previously in this section.

Triage

Triage of patients outside the ED is a quick process, less than 1 min long, to evaluate the patient and decide the severity and destination.

Critical/severe (RED) casualties are those who sustain one or more of the following life-threatening conditions:
- Respiratory distress
- Shock
- Coma/altered mental status
- Amputations

Minimal medical care is provided at the triage site:
- Ventilatory assistance with Ambu bag (if necessary)
- Tourniquets for exsanguinating limb hemorrhage

Inflow of patients:
After a brief triage, a colored chart and armbands, both matching patient severity ("Red" chart to "Red" patient) will be attached to the patients on stretchers or in wheel chairs. The transporter will then follow preestablished pathways for patient influx, identified by direction arrows on the corridor floor or walls. The selected pathway (arrow color) should match the color of the chart on the patient. This

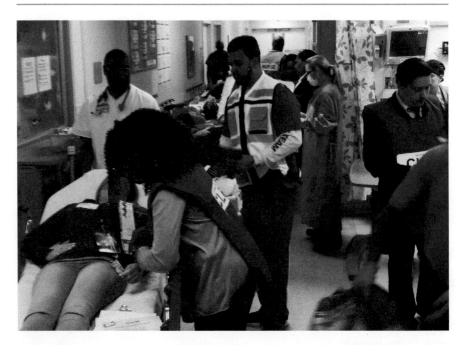

Fig. 3.15 Patient identification and registration during MCI drill, Ryder Trauma Center, Miami, 2018

system simplifies patient transport from the triage area to in-hospital treatment sites and increases the likelihood of correct patient disposition, as determined by the triage officer (Fig. 3.15).

The Medical Care Philosophy During a Sudden Mass Casualty Incident

After triage is completed, patients are distributed to the treatment sites according to the severity of injury. The medical philosophy in a SMCI is different when compared to the management of a single trauma patient.

Principles of Medical Care Inside the Treatment Sites

- Salvageable critical/severe (RED) patients are treated first!
- Traumatic injuries should be managed following ATLS® guidelines.
- The medical care for nonemergent patients should be delayed until more medical personnel become available.
- In all treatment areas, the surgeon in charge of the site or the ED physician is the one responsible for the care of the patient. All major decisions such as priorities

of care and disposition are made by the surgeon in charge of the site or ED physician (OR, radiology, ICU, or floor admission).

- No patient should leave treatment site without approval of the surgeon in charge of the site or the ED physician.
- Once the patient leaves the treatment site area, the patient does not return to the same area. Therefore, decisions regarding disposition of the patient should be made before the patient leaves the treatment site or in the radiology suite (e.g., a neurosurgeon should be in the CT scan, making immediate decisions).

Blood Bank

- Blood type and cross match (T + C) is of critical importance for the management of a trauma patient. During a SMCI, multiple requests for type and cross are expected simultaneously. Therefore, T + C is one of the two laboratory tests to be performed in the initial phase of a SMCI. The other laboratory test is arterial blood gas (see below).
- Automated systems to transport blood samples from the emergency department (ED) or trauma center (TC) maybe overwhelmed in a SMCI. Therefore, to be able to expedite transport of blood samples and avoid misidentification, "blood bank runners" should be utilized.
- The main function of the "blood bank runners" is to collect the tubes and bring them to the blood bank. They should also distribute the blood and products to the sites where needed.
- The blood bank supervisor should be in direct radio communication with sites where blood will more commonly be needed: Treatment area of the severe (RED) patients, operating room, intensive care units.
- Communication: Radio, on medical frequency, for the blood bank supervisor.

Laboratory

- Blood tests routinely performed in a single trauma patient should not be performed in a SMCI. Laboratory technicians will, most certainly, be busy performing T + C and emergency blood tests such as arterial blood gases (ABG) and hemoglobin levels.
- It will be at the discretion of the treating physician to order other tests.

Radiology

- Imaging should be scarce during the initial phase of a SMCI and limited only to examinations that will have an immediate impact on patient management.
- CXR and pelvic X-rays should be performed at the treatment site with portable X-ray units.

- Ultrasound (US) or diagnostic peritoneal lavage (DPL) should be used when intra-abdominal bleeding is suspected.
- Computerized tomography (CT) is used in the initial phase of a SMCI only for patients with suspected traumatic brain injury (Expect multiple brain CT scans to be performed in the first hours).
- Limb X-rays will only be performed for open fractures and/or for limb threatening injuries.
- Immobilization of the limb/s for clinically suspected fractures should be performed; X-rays for closed fractures should be delayed.

Family/Friends Information Center, Tracking of Patients, and Media Relations in a Sudden Mass Casualty Incident

Family/Friends Information Center (FIC) (Fig. 3.16)

There is a need to identify an area within the hospital to accommodate a sharp increase in the number of family members or friends seeking information about their loved ones. At least three family members for each patient are expected to arrive.

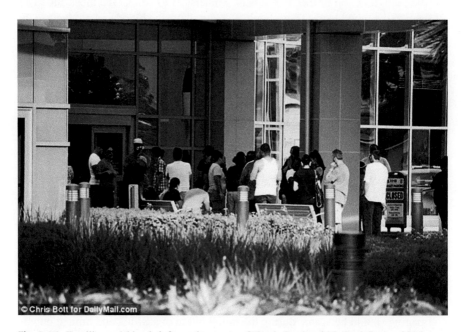

Fig. 3.16 Families and friends information center, Orlando Regional Medical Center, 2016

The basic planning of a FIC includes:
- Personnel:
  - One psychologist
  - Social workers
  - Clerks
  - Medical doctor/nurse practitioner (if available)
- Equipment:
  - Computer monitors connected to hospital information system to show pictures of unidentified patients to people searching for missing family members
- Facilities/Supplies:
  - Toilets
  - Food/drinks
  - Wi-Fi

Tracking

Tracking of patients in the community where the SMCI occurred is important and needs to be performed at the hospital level. All Israeli hospitals have one secure tracking program (ADAM) that can be accessed at any hospital in the country. Since the patients from a SMCI may be transported to any hospital in the city, this program prevents family members and friends from driving from one hospital to another in search for their loved ones. Instead, this database may be accessed at the first hospital where they arrive. If the missing family member could not be found at the first hospital, family members could then see pictures of unidentified patients at other hospitals in the city.

Prehospital tracking, although being recently tested, may be challenging in a SMCI and should not be used.

Media Center

In general, media coverage of a SMCI starts simultaneously with patient care. Reporters need a designated working area. In addition, they need to be provided with timely and updated information. A designated public relations officer of the hospital should have specific training to address the media (Fig. 3.17).

The hospital experiencing a SMCI should use the media for its own benefit: Early broadcasting of a hospital "hotline" number is of critical importance to reduce stress and anxiety of family members and friends who are eager to know the destiny of their loved ones. Media should also be used to broadcast essential instructions to the population such as evacuation routes, safety instructions, public warning, public reassurance, and the stimulation of aid and donations both locally

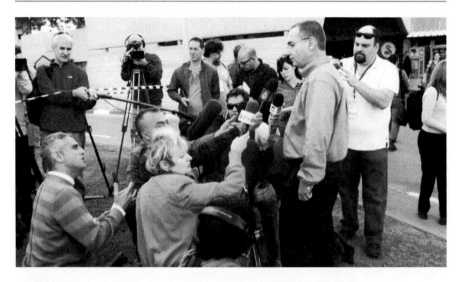

Fig. 3.17 Hospital spokesman addressing the media during a drill in Israel

and beyond. These potential benefits are instrumental in disaster management, and therefore, excellent relations between the media and medical services are essential. This is the responsibility of the public relations officer, who should use all forms of media (television, radio, print, and internet), to disseminate relevant event-related information.

Hospital Incident Command in a Sudden Mass Casualty Incident

The well-known hospital emergency incident command system (HEICS), first published in the mid-eighties, is the "brain" of the hospital during a disaster, and it provides a clear chain of command.

The structure, function, and operability of HEICS may be found elsewhere.

This chapter will discuss a different approach for a hospital incident command (HIC), which is more applicable for SMCIs.

The use of the formal HEICS is one of the best examples why the classification of disasters into progressive and sudden is important, as previously discussed.

The use of a fully deployed HEICS should be very beneficial for the hospital during a slowly developing biological epidemic, when tracking a hurricane for a few days or for a planned mass gathering such as a large open concert. In these situations, there is enough time to schedule the key personnel listed in the HEICS table of organization, while verifying that they are actually available.

Nevertheless, the use of a fully organized HEICS in a SMCI is questionable at best. Because of its unexpected nature and the fast speed of its progression, the HIC during the first hours of a SMCI should be different and include with the following features:

- Simple
- Based on the personnel on call at the hospital
- Identical for weekdays, weekends, nights, and holidays
- Mobile
- Flexible
- Expandable

As discussed in previous chapters, the initial hospital phase of the SMCI includes various stages, most of which are simultaneous:
- Preparing the triage area:
    - Deployment of stretchers, wheelchairs, medical equipment, identification and registration supplies, medical personnel, transporters, and security
- Preparing space in the emergency department (ED):
    - Outflux of patients and movement of empty stretchers to triage area
    - Absorption of additional medical and support personnel
- Preparing alternate sites of medical care:
    - Deployment of stretchers, equipment, ventilators, and supplies
    - Absorption of additional medical and support personnel
- Preparing operating rooms:
    - Scheduling surgical teams
    - Deployment of additional equipment
- Influx of patients:
    - Triage
    - Transport to treatment sites, CT scan, operating rooms, and intensive care units
    - Deployment of additional equipment and supplies to treatment areas as needed

To control all the above simultaneous stages, simplicity of a HIC is key! There is no time to wait for administrators to arrive from home; therefore, the HIC needs to be based on the on-call personnel. Since a SMCI may happen anytime, HIC needs to identical for weekdays, weekends, nights, and holidays. The mobility is critical, and the presence of the incident commander (IC), with a portable two-way radio, at the major areas of "action" is of great advantage. After visualizing the challenges, he/she may activate, through the portable communication system, any area of the hospital that is significant during the initial phase of a SMCI. Additional hospital administrators may be added to the HIC as the event progresses.

Triage Hospital

SMCIs may occur in urban areas where large Medical Centers are immediately available or in rural areas, where only small community hospitals are in proximity. A good example is a train derailment outside major urban areas (Fig. 3.18).

"Triage hospital" is a concept not an actual building. This concept was developed for small community hospitals that are the closest medical facility to the SMCI. These

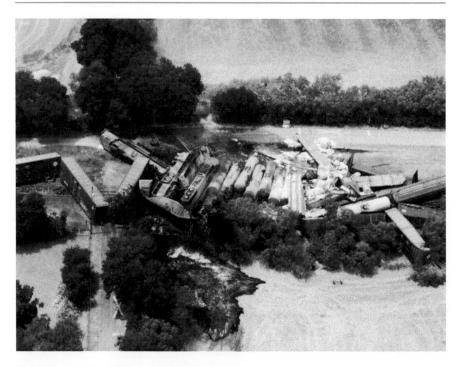

Fig. 3.18 Train derailment in Macdona, Texas, 2004

smaller rural hospitals typically lack major surgical specialties such as neurosurgery, burns, and cardio-thoracic surgery.

Since it is the only medical facility in the area, ambulances may by default transport patients to this hospital.

In principle, a "triage hospital" functions as "resuscitation hospital." It performs all necessary procedures to stabilize the injured patient, including surgery for hemorrhage control, when indicated.

All patients, after initial stabilization, are transferred to higher level medical facilities. Patients who underwent emergency surgery, will remain at the community hospital until their condition is stabilized and then transferred to higher level hospitals.

The switch of a community medical center from being an admitting hospital into a "triage hospital" requires a declaration by the hospital's CEO and communication to the regional emergency operation center.

The concept of a "triage hospital" should be part of the Regional Disaster Plan.

Medical Challenges in Managing Blast Injuries

4

Mauricio Lynn

Introduction

This is not another chapter about blast injuries but rather a brief summary of the main challenges encountered when treating patients with these catastrophic injuries.

Classification of Blast Injuries

- *Primary:* It is related to the impact of the blast wave (pressure wave) on the body.
  - Damages usually occur in air containing organs:
  - Tympanic membrane.
  - Upper and lower airways.
  - Lungs (Fig. 4.1).
  - Intestine.

It also may affect solid organs:

- Heart (contusions, hemorrhages, air embolism, acute myocardial infarction, cor pulmonale) (Fig. 4.2).
- Brain (contusion, contrecoup, hemorrhage, air embolism).
- Extremities (blast amputations).
- *Secondary:* Injuries caused by shrapnel.
  - Usually penetrating injuries to torso and/or extremities (Fig. 4.3).
- *Tertiary:* IT is related to the "landing of the victim" after being pushed by the blast wave and blast wind.
  - Penetrating injuries if patients lands of sharp objects (Fig. 4.4).
  - Blunt trauma if patient lands on concrete or ground.

M. Lynn
University of Miami Miller School of Medicine, Jackson Memorial Hospital,
Department of Surgery, Miami, FL, USA
e-mail: mlynn@med.miami.edu

© Springer Nature Switzerland AG 2019
M. Lynn et al. (eds.), *Disasters and Mass Casualty Incidents*,
https://doi.org/10.1007/978-3-319-97361-6_4

Fig. 4.1 Pulmonary blast
injury

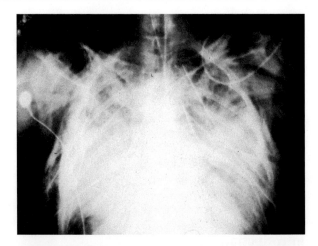

Fig. 4.2 Postmortem
image showing heart and
lungs hemorrhagic
contusions following blast

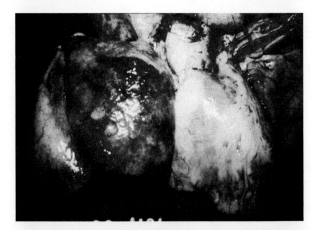

Fig. 4.3 Secondary blast
injury: nail penetrating
extremity

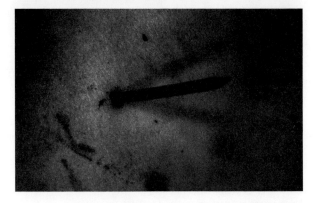

Fig. 4.4 Tertiary blast injury: patient "landed" on a piece of glass

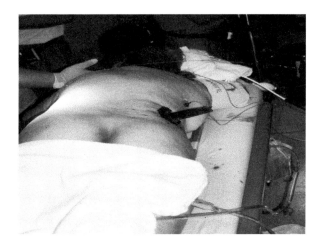

Fig. 4.5 "Multidimensional" injury: combination of all types of blast injuries simultaneously

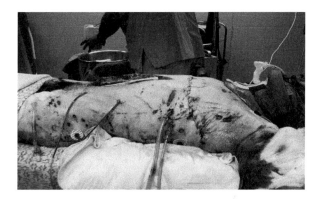

- *Quaternary:* Injuries related by the heat of the explosion, known as "flash burns," usually affecting exposed areas such as scalp, face, neck, and uncovered extremities.
- *Multidimensional:* It was proposed recently by Israeli physicians to describe patients who present will all types of blast injuries simultaneously and the potential of viral exposure from infected body parts (bones) of suicide bombers ("secondary shrapnel") (Fig. 4.5).

The main challenges facing medical personnel when managing patients with blast injuries:
- Ruling out "hidden" internal injuries in walking wounded patients:
  - Perform ear exam on all suspected patients. Presence of an intact tympanic membrane most likely rules out internal injuries. (Fig. 4.6).
- Management of severe pulmonary blast injury and prevention of air embolism:
  - Position of patients: Prone or left lateral, and Trendelenburg.
  - Ventilatory support: Preferably noninvasive or low pressure, using high supplemental oxygen, may consider nitric oxide.

Fig. 4.6 Ruptured
tympanic membrane
following explosion

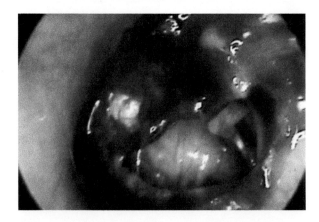

- Considering early extra corporeal membrane oxygenation (ECMO) for severe pulmonary hemorrhage.
- Fluids: Maintain normovolemia.
- Considering hyperbaric therapy for air embolism.
- Early decompressive laparotomy for abdominal compartment syndrome.
• Management of cardiac complications from primary blast injuries:
- Standard care for acute myocardial infarction (AMI) due to air embolism to coronaries, considering hyperbaric therapy.
- Standard management for pulmonary heart disease (cor pulmonale) from pulmonary embolism and severe acute respiratory distress syndrome.
• Management of neurologic complications from primary blast injuries:
- Standard care for brain injury caused by brain contusion, contrecoup, hemorrhage.
- Considering hyperbaric therapy for brain air embolism.
• Management of "multidimensional" blast injury:
- Priorities of care, for simultaneous blast injuries, by following ATLS® guidelines.
- Immunoglobulin administration for "secondary shrapnel".

Medical Aspects of Volcanic Eruptions

5

Bradley S. Moffat

Volcanic eruptions are relatively rare occurring natural disasters. In the past century, there have been 27 volcanic eruptions resulting in fatalities worldwide. While most volcanic events have limited casualties, owing to advanced warning and preparedness in high-risk zones, eruptions may sometimes be sudden and occur in densely populated areas where mass casualties and mass fatalities can be catastrophic. The most lethal volcanic eruption in modern history occurred in Nevado del Ruiz, Columbia in 1985 killing over 23,000 and injuring over 10,000 (Fig. 5.1).

Volcanoes produce unique geological phenomena that can injure or kill large groups of people living in the vicinity. Pyroclastic flows are superheated plumes of gas and debris that flow with great speed out of an erupting volcano like an avalanche. These events can produce *severe burns* as well as *direct trauma* as they progress and can travel for 100 km or more before they dissipate. Lava flows can also be extremely destructive but usually flow relatively slowly and, therefore, represent low risk to human life. Debris flows called "lahars" can be generated as large amounts of snow, ice, and mud are melted during an eruption leading to vast, fast-moving flows which often concentrate in valleys where humans are situated. Lahars can cause extreme damage and death along their paths. Eruptions produce massive amounts of ejecta including ash and particulate matter which is collectively known as "tephra." Tephra can be inhaled causing *respiratory problems* and can also accumulate on roads leading to traffic accidents or on structures leading to collapse. It can hamper rescue efforts by cutting off access to disaster areas both by blocking roads and preventing air travel as was demonstrated by the Icelandic eruption of Eyjafjallajökull in 2010 which grounded air travel in the area for weeks. Hazardous gases can also be ejected during eruptions which include sulfur dioxide, sulfuric acid, hydrochloric acid, hydrogen sulfide, mercury, and radon.

B. S. Moffat
Jackson Memorial Hospital, Ryder Trauma Center, Miami, FL, USA
e-mail: bradley.moffat@jhsmiami.org

© Springer Nature Switzerland AG 2019
M. Lynn et al. (eds.), *Disasters and Mass Casualty Incidents*,
https://doi.org/10.1007/978-3-319-97361-6_5

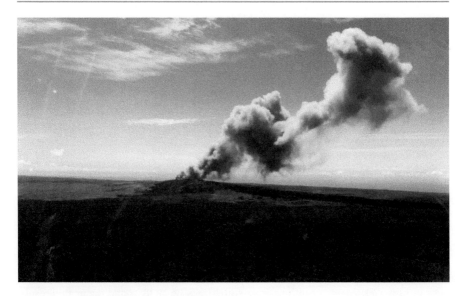

Fig. 5.1 Volcanic eruption, Hawaii, 2018

One of the major barriers during volcano response is accessing the victims. While some may be able to self-evacuate, the extreme destruction brought on by an eruption will hinder both egress of walking wounded and access of rescue teams. Unfortunately, this delay often results in the most severely injured survivors dying from their injuries or other volcano related hazards before they can be evacuated to hospital. However, for those that do survive, it may take days or weeks to rescue them and responding teams and hospitals should expect increased flow of patients throughout this process.

Most common injuries after volcanic eruption:

- Direct blunt trauma due to the following reasons:
  - Falling ejecta.
  - Lahars.
  - Pyroclastic flows.
  - Motor vehicle crashes due to ash on roads.
- Eye irritation.
- Compounding problems:
  - Burns.
  - Respiratory diseases.
  - Hazardous materials exposure.

Although respiratory problems are surprisingly minor among survivors, *Ash asphyxiation* is one of the leading causes of death among volcano fatalities. To date, there have been no measurable long-term respiratory problems attributed to volcanic eruptions.

Pyroclastic flows were once thought to represent a nonsurvivable phenomenon. Indeed pyroclastic flows alone account for over one third of all volcano-related deaths. Several studies, however, have demonstrated that some burn patients do survive pyroclastic flows and can be expected to reach hospital needing treatment. A recent study examining the pyroclastic flows resulting from the 1994 and 2010 eruptions of the Merapi volcano in Java looked at 106 burn patients. Almost 80% of the burn patients presented with more than 40% of total body surface area burned. Most of these burn patients also had inhalational injury. About a third of the burn patients survived their hospitalization.

It is estimated that less than 5% of volcano survivors will present with illness related to hazardous gas exposure.

Burns Mass Casualty Incident

6

Mauricio Lynn and Nicholas Namias

Burns and thermal injuries are common in sudden mass casualty incidents (SMCIs) associated with explosions and fires (Figs. 6.1 and 6.2) and may present in the form of radiation, chemical, or flame burns. In addition, all types of burns may be associated with inhalation of fumes or vapor that further damages the airway and lungs.

Principles of triage of burn patients during a SMCI follow the same triage criteria as discussed previously, and the initial management follows the Advanced Trauma Life Support (ATLS)® and Advanced Burn Life Support (ABLS)® guidelines for burn patients, with or without combined traumatic injuries.

Nevertheless, management of a burn mass casualty incident (BMCI) has specific challenges:

- Fluid resuscitation should be performed following the American burn association (ABA) consensus formula, which is the most commonly used method for calculation of the amount of fluids to be infused.
- The formula: 2–4 cc/Kg/%BSA per 24 h. Half the amount is infused in the first 8 h. After a first few hours, fluids should be titrated according to hourly urinary output.
- Excision and grafting of burns is not an emergency procedure and may be initiated within a week from the injury. Therefore, in a BMCI, protection of the burns with silver-based creams or dressings is considered adequate care in the acute phase of the event.
- There is no need for specialized equipment and supplies for the initial management of a BMCI in emergency departments (ED) or trauma centers (TC).
- Trauma surgeons and emergency medicine physicians should be able to manage the initial resuscitation and care of a burn patient prior to transfer to a burn unit, if needed.

M. Lynn (✉) · N. Namias
University of Miami Miller School of Medicine, Jackson Memorial Hospital,
Department of Surgery, Miami, FL, USA
e-mail: mlynn@med.miami.edu

© Springer Nature Switzerland AG 2019
M. Lynn et al. (eds.), *Disasters and Mass Casualty Incidents*,
https://doi.org/10.1007/978-3-319-97361-6_6

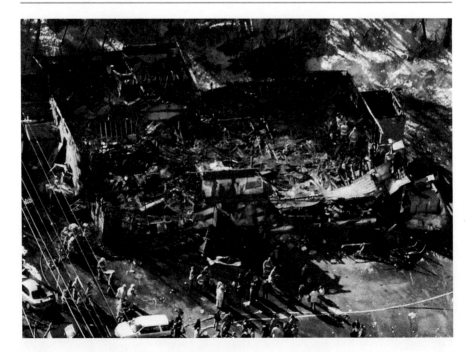

Fig. 6.1 Nightclub fire, Rhode Island, US, 2003

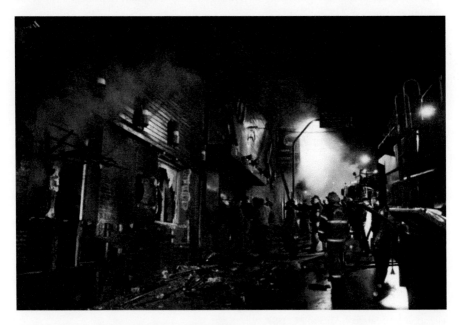

Fig. 6.2 Nightclub fire, Santa Maria, Brazil, 2013

- The injuries and resuscitation may lead to compartment syndromes (discussed later in this section) that require emergency decompression by escharotomy and/or fasciotomy. General or orthopedic surgeons should be able to perform this procedure.
- Criteria for transfer of burn injuries to a burn center that are relevant to a BMCI, include as follows:
  - Partial thickness burns greater than 20% total body surface area (TBSA).
    - Note: When not in a SMCI situation, the criteria for transfer are partial thickness burns greater than 10% total TBSA.
  - Burns that involve the face, hands, feet, genitalia, perineum, or major joints.
  - Third degree burns in any age group.
  - Electrical burns, including lightning injury.
  - Chemical burns.
  - Inhalation injury.
  - Burn injury in patients with preexisting medical disorders that could complicate management, prolong recovery, or affect mortality.
  - Burned children in hospitals without qualified personnel or equipment for the care of children.
  - Any patient with burns and concomitant trauma (such as fractures) in which the burn injury poses the greatest risk of morbidity or mortality.
  - If the traumatic injuries pose greater immediate risk, the patient should be initially stabilized in a TC/ED before being transferred to a burn unit.
  - Physician judgment will be necessary in such situations and should be in concert with the regional emergency operations center and triage protocols during a SMCI.
- Transfer of a large number of burn patients to burn centers simultaneously may require air resources such as helicopters and fixed wing airplanes, and may present huge logistical challenges.

Medical Response to Mass Shootings

7

Bradley S. Moffat

Epidemiology

Although mass shootings have occurred for decades, the Columbine High School shooting in 1999 marked a pivotal turning point on the understanding, anticipation, and preparedness for mass shooting events. Between Columbine and the more recent mass shootings in Las Vegas and Parkland, Florida (2017 and 2018, respectively), there have been over 70 mass shooting events in the United States. A total of 620 people have been killed, and over 1000 people have been wounded. The deadliest mass shooting in US history occurred in October 2017 when a lone gunman armed with multiple assault rifles opened fire on a music festival, killing 58 and wounding 546 people (Fig. 7.1).

A mass shooting is generally defined as an incident where 3–5 people are intentionally shot in the same event.

Important aspects to consider when preparing to respond to as mass shooting incident:

- Pattern of injury among survivors.
- Cause of death among fatalities.
- Timeline of the event.

B. S. Moffat
Jackson Memorial Hospital, Ryder Trauma Center, Miami, FL, USA
e-mail: bradley.moffat@jhsmiami.org

© Springer Nature Switzerland AG 2019
M. Lynn et al. (eds.), *Disasters and Mass Casualty Incidents*,
https://doi.org/10.1007/978-3-319-97361-6_7

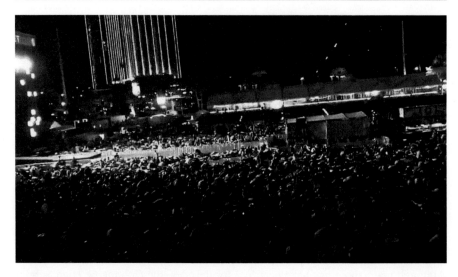

Fig. 7.1 Mass shooting in Las Vegas, US, 2017

Prehospital

Triage of victims:
- Identify *critical and salvageable* patients.
- Perform life-saving maneuvers:
  - Open airway.
  - Needle thoracostomy to relieve tension pneumothorax.
  - Bleeding control in extremities.
- Recognize victims with nonsurvivable injuries.
- Victims with *absent vital signs* should be tagged as expectant and *not* be transported to hospital.

Note: A study from George Washington University (Arlington, VA) looked at the pattern of wounding for 139 mass shooting fatalities from 12 different mass shooting events. 58% of patients had injuries to the head or chest, and these injuries constituted the probable fatal wounds in 77% of cases. Among victims who died, only 7% had potentially survivable injuries with almost all of these injuries being gunshot wounds to the chest. *None of the patients died from extremity hemorrhage.*

Although there has been a recent emphasis on controlling extremity hemorrhage immediately in the field during mass shooting events, it is interesting to note that exsanguination from extremity gunshot wound was not identified as the fatal wound for any of the victims in the George Washington University study. The American College of Surgeons has developed a campaign titled "Stop the Bleed." This campaign focuses on early application of tourniquets by bystanders to stop extremity hemorrhage, with a focus on mass shooting events. While early control of major bleeding from extremity gunshots wounds is desired, the risks to civilians, when the scene is not yet cleared by law enforcement, must be weighed against the evidence showing that very few victims of mass shootings die from extremity hemorrhage.

Emergency Department

A critical factor to consider when planning for mass shooting events is the timing of egress of patients from the scene.

As discussed previously in this book, the first victims to arrive at the ED after a sudden mass casualty incident (SMCI) will be the walking wounded and the self-evacuees ("Chaos phase"). These patients are likely to be transported before a formal incident command is set up and before scene triage has been initiated. This was acutely displayed during the "Pulse" nightclub shooting in Orlando, Florida in 2016. The first wave arrived within minutes (Fig. 7.2).

Hospital personnel should be aware of this phenomenon and *not* load the ED with walking-wounded victims before better information from the scene becomes available. Most likely, the critical victims will arrive in the second wave.

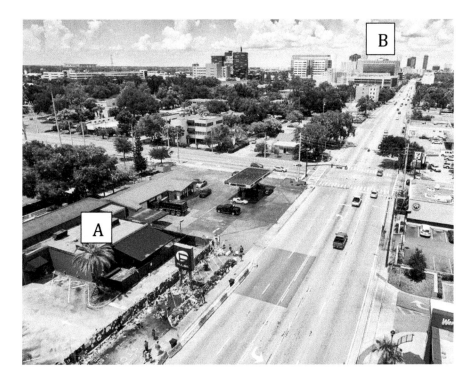

Fig. 7.2 Short distance between "Pulse" nightclub (**A**) and Orlando Regional Medical Center (**B**)

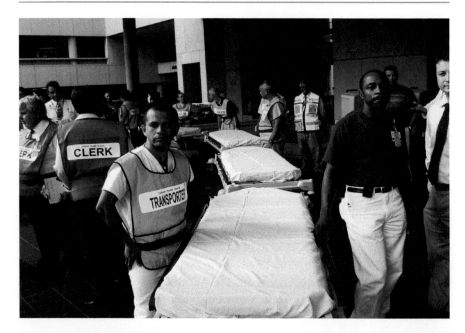

Fig. 7.3 Triage area at Jackson Memorial Hospital, Miami, FL, ready to receive victims during a simulation for SMCI

Unfortunately, in Orlando, the second wave did not arrive at Orlando Regional Medical Center (ORMC) until 3 h after the shooting began, as there was a hostage situation at the club and the shooter could not be suppressed during a long period of time (Fig. 7.3).

When receiving patients from a mass shooting event or any other SMCI, surgeons should not perform resuscitative thoracotomies, especially in those with gunshot wounds to the head or torso. The survival rate for these patients is near zero, and resources are likely to be needed for other patients arriving later in the course of the event. This represents an important shift from the standard resuscitative thoracotomy performed in a single patient, in arrest, from a gunshot wound to the torso.

Anticipating emergency OR needs is an important part of planning for mass shooting disasters. Unlike other SMCIs, mass shootings have a relatively increased proportion of victims requiring immediate life-saving surgery (for hemostasis) and urgent operations. It is anticipated that about two thirds of mass shooting victims may require surgery. Therefore, there is a need to have one or two operating rooms (ORs) immediately available for life-saving surgery. While more OR staff is called in, other rooms are made available for the urgent cases, typically within 1 or 2 h. As the hospital response escalates over time, additional operating rooms should be made available for the less urgent surgeries to be completed.

Use of Tourniquets in Mass Casualty Incidents and "Stop the Bleed" Program

8

Mauricio Lynn

Introduction

- The use of tourniquets, as a temporary procedure to control extremity bleeding, may be life saving.
- For many years, the use of tourniquets was banned from civilian prehospital protocols for management of limb hemorrhage due to concerns for complications, mainly loss of limbs.
- Military studies published by the Israeli, Americans, and British in the past 15 years, show that tourniquets are effective to control bleeding in the battlefield, are associated with minor complications and no limb loss.
- These outcomes were replicated in civilian studies as well. Recently, the advanced trauma life support (ATLS®) course introduced tourniquet use as an alternative for management of limb hemorrhage, when direct pressure fails to control bleeding.
- Nevertheless, in some situations when improvised tourniquets (cloths, ropes, ties) are applied by untrained bystanders, the opposite effect may occur, and the bleeding may increase.
- Therefore, tourniquet application should be limited to trained personnel. Untrained bystanders should be allowed to hold pressure directly on the bleeding site until trained personnel arrive.
- The "Stop the Bleed" training program, recently introduced by the American College of Surgeons (ACS), should increase the number of bystanders trained to control the bleeding until EMS arrives.

M. Lynn
University of Miami Miller School of Medicine, Jackson Memorial Hospital,
Department of Surgery, Miami, FL, USA
e-mail: mlynn@med.miami.edu

© Springer Nature Switzerland AG 2019
M. Lynn et al. (eds.), *Disasters and Mass Casualty Incidents*,
https://doi.org/10.1007/978-3-319-97361-6_8

Indications for Tourniquet Placement

- Failure of direct pressure to control the bleeding.
- Multiple bleeding sites on the same limb/s where direct pressure is not feasible (Fig. 8.1).
- Bleeding stump after traumatic amputation.
- Need for airway management and hemorrhage control simultaneously by ONE provider.
- Long walking evacuation from the scene to an ambulance/helicopter.
- Mass casualty incident, with multiple bleeding patients and few providers.

Application of Tourniquets

- It is very difficult if not impossible, even for an experienced EMS provider, to distinguish between arterial and venous bleeding, mainly in low light situations.
- Therefore, a tourniquet should be always placed above (proximal) to the bleeding site.
- The tourniquet should be tightened until bleeding stops or is reduced significantly.
- A pressure dressing should be applied as well, to reduce small oozing.
- Patient should be immediately transported to a trauma center (Fig. 8.2).

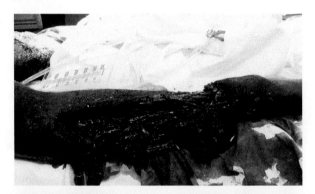

Fig. 8.1 Mangled extremity where direct pressure is not feasible

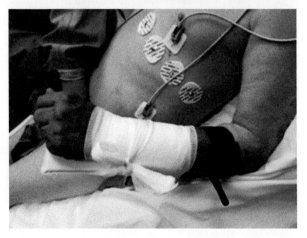

Fig. 8.2 Tourniquet applied by EMS and transported to Ryder Trauma Center, Miami, FL

Removal of Tourniquet at the Trauma Center

• Resuscitation of the patient at the trauma center should follow ATLS® guidelines.
• Prior to removal of the tourniquet, the patient should be assessed for associated injuries.
• Two large bore IVs should be inserted and blood available prior tourniquet removal.
• If after removal of the tourniquet, the bleeding appears to be less than initially thought, pressure dressing should be applied.
• If after removal of the tourniquet, the bleeding appears to be brisk, direct pressure should be attempted. If bleeding is severe, tourniquet should be reapplied and patient managed according to trauma principles.
• If patient has associated torso injuries that require immediate hemostasis, tourniquet may be kept in place until thoracotomy/laparotomy is completed (Fig. 8.3).

"Stop the Bleed" Program

• "Buddy aid" is a military concept where a soldier is trained to assist an injured soldier, including hemorrhage control, until the unit medic is available to take over the care.
• Launched by the White House in October 2015 and adopted by the ACS, the "Stop the Bleed" program is meant to replicate the "buddy aid" concept and encourage bystanders to become trained, equipped, and empowered to help in a bleeding emergency before professional help arrives.
• In contrast to the soldier, the bystander is not equipped with protective gear such as helmet, bullet proof vests, and does not carry a weapon for self-defense.

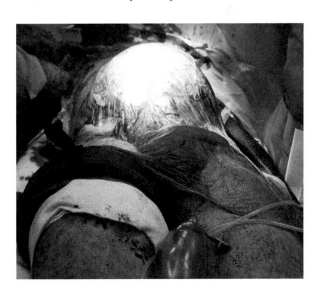

Fig. 8.3 Tourniquet remained in place until laparotomy was completed for combined torso and limb injuries

- In addition, a study from George Washington University in 2015 looked at the pattern of wounding for 139 fatalities from 12 different mass shooting events. None of the patients died from extremity hemorrhage.
- Trained bystanders should be encouraged to help injured friends and other citizens when the scene is pronounced "clear" by law enforcement agencies.
- Attempts to assist, prior to scene control by law enforcement, may increase the number of victims by the presence of an active shooter or secondary devices.

Psychological Considerations in the Aftermath of School Sudden Mass Casualty Incidents

Lauren Zakaib

When shooting occurs at schools, a chaos phase transpires within the school setting. It is important that every school district has an updated *crisis manual* to outline particular procedures, to reduce the severity of the chaos period. Once the first responders, such as fireman, policeman, and paramedics, address and stabilize the injured students and faculty, then the mental health first responders step in. Mental health services following a sudden mass casualty incident (SMCI) within the school is critical because it has the possibility to decrease the likelihood of further psychological trauma. Every school should have a designated crisis leader, preferably with mental health background.

Although students and staff may not have been physically injured, those in close proximity of the incident (bystander trauma) can demonstrate characteristics associated with post-traumatic stress disorder (PTSD). In addition to physical proximity, PTSD can also have profound effects on individuals within a close emotional proximity with the victims (e.g., best friend, teacher, tutor). Childhood trauma can increase the risk for psychological, behavioral, or emotional problems (depression or PTSD), substance abuse, low occupational attainment or academic failure, social maladjustment, and poor medical health.

After a SMCI occurs:
- A designated crisis leader should be assigned and:
  - Organize the counseling services.
  - Address safety measures.
  - Handle media involvement.

L. Zakaib
Psychological Services, Broward County School District, Fort Lauderdale, FL, USA

© Springer Nature Switzerland AG 2019
M. Lynn et al. (eds.), *Disasters and Mass Casualty Incidents*,
https://doi.org/10.1007/978-3-319-97361-6_9

- A school-based crisis response team should be prepared to begin crisis counseling immediately or the following day. Crisis response team members within the school setting should consist of:
  - School psychologists.
  - Social workers.
  - Counselors.

Crisis response team members should be trained in crisis counseling and debriefed of the event. It is important to note when providing services within the school setting, individuals must be cleared to work with the students. This can vary by school district; however, it is best to assemble a team within district personal that has been cleared to work with students (e.g., school badge, finger printed, and background check).

- A designated counseling location, also known as a "psychological triage," should be assigned to provide counseling services (e.g., community center and recreation center) to students, staff, and parents. After a school shooting, services should not be provided within the school setting until the building has been restored (e.g., bullet holes fixed, blood cleaned). Throughout this critical time following a SMCI, students need to feel safe.
  - Additional community resources can be provided at the center.
  - Service dogs, in addition to counseling, can be helpful in the therapeutic process.

Crisis Response Brief Checklist for SMCI

- Immediately report to designated site of crisis counseling.
- Report location change to regional/district office.
- Check in with the crisis team manager.
- Prepare psychological triage with water, snacks, and tissues.
- Support in the development of a crisis response plan with the team.
  - Create designated sections for individual- and small-group counseling locations.
  - Pair up two crisis responders to hold group counseling sessions together.
- Provide counseling support.
  - In addition, provide handouts and resources to help individuals cope during the distressing time.
- Maintain logs of students seen in counseling with notes regarding follow-up recommendations.
- Engage in debriefing session with the crisis team at the end of the day.
- Assess evolving needs and participate in the development of the crisis plan for the next day.
- Participate in self-care activities when not scheduled to work.
  - The adults providing support to affected students may experience difficulties themselves. These adults will need support in learning to manage their own reactions and stress.

Planning the Medical Response to Earthquakes

10

Mauricio Lynn

Introduction

The major distinction between planning the medical response to earthquakes and other sudden mass casualty incidents (SMCI) is related to how severe damage will be the infrastructure of the city where the earthquake occurred.

There is a high possibility that roads, airports, communications, and hospitals will be partially or completely damaged, which will significantly delay search and rescue efforts, transportation of sick or injured, medical care, and outcome of victims.

Epidemiology of Earthquakes

Some distinct clusters of medical problems should be expected after an earthquake:
- Traumatic and crush injuries: Occur as a result of building collapse.
- Burn injuries: Occur from fires, boiling water, or steam, as a result damaged infrastructure.
- Near drowning: Occur as a result of flooding.
- Infectious diseases: As a result of simultaneous damage to sewage and water systems.
- Respiratory diseases: As a result of huge amount of dust from collapsed buildings/ homes.
- Radiation contamination: As a result of nuclear meltdown after damage to local nuclear reactor (Fig. 10.1).

M. Lynn
University of Miami Miller School of Medicine, Jackson Memorial Hospital,
Department of Surgery, Miami, FL, USA
e-mail: mlynn@med.miami.edu

© Springer Nature Switzerland AG 2019
M. Lynn et al. (eds.), *Disasters and Mass Casualty Incidents*,
https://doi.org/10.1007/978-3-319-97361-6_10

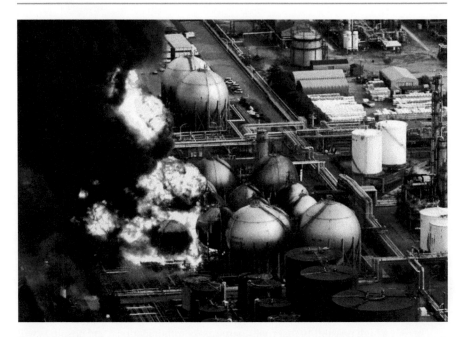

Fig. 10.1 Fukushima nuclear reactor after earthquake and tsunami, Japan, 2011

Rapid Assessment

It is of critical importance to perform an immediate rapid assessment of the area affected by the earthquake and decide if external help is needed.
- Use helicopters for rapid assessment
- Assess the extent of damage:
  - Disruption of communication: Cell towers, power lines, telephone lines
  - Disruption of transport: Roads, rails, airport (Fig. 10.2)
- Assess damage to hospitals:
  - Total collapse
  - Partial collapse
  - Electrical power
- Assessment team critical needs:
  - Helicopters
  - Satellite communications
  - Temporary incident command structure for early important decisions.
  - Request external help *early*

Search and Rescue techniques can be found in a separate chapter in this section.

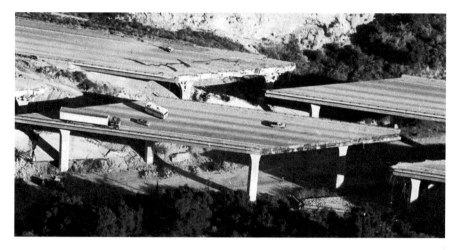

Fig. 10.2 Damage to interstate after Northridge earthquake, California, 1994

Medical Care

- The medical resources, hospitals and personnel, may be insufficient to provide optimal medical care to all survivors.
- Five levels of medical care may need to be provided to survivors:
  - Immediate first aid
  - Advanced trauma life support (ATLS®) for traumatic, crush injuries and burns
  - Resuscitative surgery mainly for hemostasis and completion of amputations.
  - Field anesthesia and analgesia
  - Intensive care for critical trauma patients, near drowning, respiratory failure due to inhalation of smoke and dust
- The biggest dilemma is to decide which patients will receive what level of care in face of large numbers of patients, collapsed hospitals, and scarce medical personnel and supplies.
- This is the best time to provide the *best possible medical care to the greatest number of patients.*
- Additional challenges occur after about a week when earthquake-related injuries decrease significantly. Nevertheless, normal pattern of diseases seen in emergency departments will start to accumulate and will seek medical attention (Fig. 10.3).

Hospital out of function

- A rapid engineering assessment is of critical importance to decide whether the hospital is functional or partially or completely out of function.
- Areas to be assessed:
  - Electricity
  - Generators

Fig. 10.3 Patterns of
injuries after an earthquake

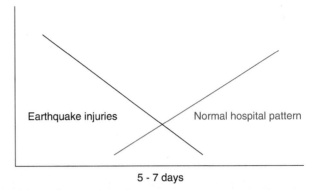

Earthquake injuries   Normal hospital pattern

5 - 7 days

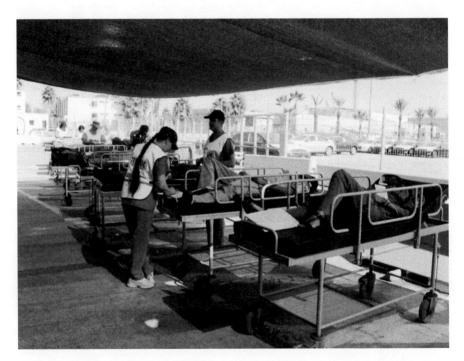

Fig. 10.4 Provision of out-of-hospital medical care during an earthquake drill in Israel

- – Elevators
- – Stairways
- Major ethical challenges will need to be addressed regarding life and death decisions of critical patients that cannot be evacuated from hospitals due to damaged
  elevators and stairways or cannot be treated locally because of lack of resources
  and transportation.
- This will require the establishment of a hospital ethical committee to evaluate
  and discuss all critical patients and decide their plan of care.
- It is possible to open medical facilities outside the damaged hospital, at the adjacent campus, and utilize intact equipment and supplies. ATLS® will probably be
  the highest level of care to be provided in such a situation (Fig. 10.4).

Search and Rescue Techniques in the Aftermath of Earthquakes

11

Mauricio Lynn

Introduction

Search and rescue (S&R) need to start as early as possible. Possibility of finding survivors beneath the rubble is directly proportional to time (Fig. 11.1).

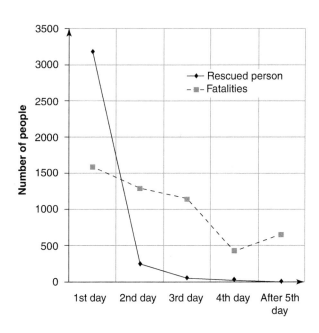

Fig. 11.1 Demonstration of the importance of early S&R after earthquakes

M. Lynn
University of Miami Miller School of Medicine, Jackson Memorial Hospital,
Department of Surgery, Miami, FL, USA
e-mail: mlynn@med.miami.edu

© Springer Nature Switzerland AG 2019
M. Lynn et al. (eds.), *Disasters and Mass Casualty Incidents*,
https://doi.org/10.1007/978-3-319-97361-6_11

Search and Rescue Techniques

- Educating the population that live in areas prone to earthquakes, on how to extricate fellow citizens, is of critical importance. Approximately 3000 (80%) of 3600 earthquake survivors in Italy are alive because they were extricated by other survivors.
- Rescue dogs: These highly trained dogs are commonly used to find survivors beneath the rubble.
- Miniature audio and video equipment: This type of fiber optic equipment is inserted beneath the rubbles to listen to faint voices, breath sounds, or to visualize trapped survivors.
- Thermal technology: This sophisticated equipment is able to locate heat sources beneath the rubble assuming the survivor can still produce body heat.
- Local knowledge: It is important to get assistance from locals and neighbors who may know the people who live in the collapsed structure.

   Safety considerations for the S&R crews:
- The structure of all buildings in an earthquake area is unstable until proven otherwise.
- Presence of a civil engineer as part of the S&R team is of vital importance.
- Entering a damaged building and dislodging already collapsed pieces of cement or stones, prior to clearance by engineering experts, may cause further injuries and death among the rescuers.
- It is imperative to use protective gear, such as helmet, eye protection goggles, dust mask, gloves when entering a partially collapsed structure.

Management of Crush Injuries and Crush Syndrome

12

Mauricio Lynn

Definitions

Crush injury – Occurs as a result of *pressure* applied to any part of the body, usually extremities, for a prolonged period of time. It may be associated or not with limb fractures. Complications of a crush injury are *crush syndrome* and *compartment syndrome.*

Compartment syndrome – Occurs as a result of increased pressure inside the limb compartments, upper or lower, and may lead to loss of limb or life, if not diagnosed and treated early.

The diagnosis of compartment syndrome are based on the following clinical signs and symptoms:

- Pain. Usually out of proportion compared to the injury. It is usually an early symptom.
- Poikilothermia.
- Paresthesia.
- Paresis.
- Pallor.
- Pulselessness.

1

M. Lynn
University of Miami Miller School of Medicine, Jackson Memorial Hospital,
Department of Surgery, Miami, FL, USA
e-mail: mlynn@med.miami.edu

© Springer Nature Switzerland AG 2019
M. Lynn et al. (eds.), *Disasters and Mass Casualty Incidents*,
https://doi.org/10.1007/978-3-319-97361-6_12

Crush syndrome – is the systemic manifestations of the crush injury and include as follows:

- Metabolic abnormalities:
  - Acidosis
  - Hyperkalemia
  - Hypocalcemia
- Renal failure

Challenges

Management of trapped victim at the scene, prior to rescue:
- Large amount of fluids: 1–1.5 liter/h during extrication.
- Consider administration of bicarbonate.
- Consider tourniquet application to limb prior to extraction.
- May need limb amputation to be able to extricate.
  - Requires transport of a trauma surgeon and anesthesiologist to the scene.

Management of patient immediately after extrication and at hospital
- Large amount of fluids until urinary output >300 cc/h.
- Correct acidosis, hyperkalemia, and hypocalcemia.
- Consider mannitol in addition to fluids in attempt to prevent renal failure.
- Renal failure may need dialysis.
- May require fasciotomy for limb compartment syndrome.

Part II

Non-conventional Sudden Mass Casualty Incidents

Introduction

This section will focus on the medical organization required to manage non-conventional events of sudden onset, such as chemical contamination or radiation exposure.

Decontamination for Chemical Exposure: At the Scene or at the Hospital?

13

Mauricio Lynn

One of the major controversies on prehospital care for sudden chemical mass casualty incidents (SCMCIs) is whether to perform mass decontamination at the scene or at the hospital.

Common chemical agents that require decontamination after exposure:

- Organophosphates
- Mustards

Epidemiology

The vast majority of the patients exposed to a chemical agent, such as an organophosphate, will be mildly contaminated ("walking wounded").

Lessons learned from the Sarin gas attack in Tokyo subway (Fig. 13.1):

- 82% of patients that arrived at medical centers in the city were self-evacuated or transported by other citizens.
- 25% of the hospital staffs at local hospitals were contaminated.

In a scenario of a SCMCI, where decontamination may be needed, there are two options:

M. Lynn
University of Miami Miller School of Medicine, Jackson Memorial Hospital,
Department of Surgery, Miami, FL, USA
e-mail: mlynn@med.miami.edu

© Springer Nature Switzerland AG 2019
M. Lynn et al. (eds.), *Disasters and Mass Casualty Incidents*,
https://doi.org/10.1007/978-3-319-97361-6_13

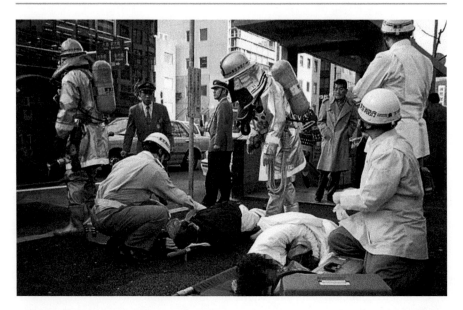

Fig. 13.1 Sarin gas attack, Tokyo, Japan, 1995

Decontamination at the Scene

- Preferable because it decreases decontamination duration and decreases risk to hospital personnel when patients arrive at the hospitals.
- Nevertheless, the time to set up decontamination capability at the scene is too long, and it is doubtful the "walking wounded," which are the vast majority, will actually wait to be decontaminated. In addition, by the time decontamination is available, most critical patients, with respiratory failure, will probably expire. Therefore, these patients should be transported rapidly to hospitals with mass decontamination capabilities by first responders with personal protective equipment (PPE).
- However, simple steps such as removal of clothing from exposed individuals, if done quickly after exposure, may reduce the contamination by 80–90%.

Decontamination at the Hospital

If a hospital has a large preprepared decontamination area, it is preferable to decontaminate at the hospital, for the reasons below:
- Most patients will self-evacuate to the hospital.
- The decontamination area could be activated within minutes from notification.

- There should be enough trained staff and personnel to handle the event.
- In addition to decontamination, patients will receive adequate medications and antidotes, which may be lacking at the scene.

Note Decontamination at the hospital carries the risk of contamination of hospital personnel. Nevertheless, this risk should be minimized if the hospital is equipped with adequate personal protective equipment (PPE) and has performed enough training and drills.

Hospital Planning and Response for Sudden Chemical Mass Casualty Incidents

Mauricio Lynn

Assumptions

- Sudden exposure of multiple people to a chemical agent may be classified as a sudden chemical mass casualty incident (SCMCI).
- The vast majority of the contaminated patients will be mildly contaminated ("walking wounded").
- The majority of contaminated patients will self-evacuate or be transported by nonrescue personnel to local hospitals.
- Although decontamination at the scene is desirable, it is time consuming in an unplanned, sudden event, and therefore unrealistic.
- Most critical patients, usually those with respiratory distress, will probably expire by the time scene decontamination is available. Therefore, critical contaminated patients should be transported rapidly to hospitals by first responders who must have personal protective equipment (PPE). Removal of all clothing may reduce contamination by 80–90% and should be done prior to getting into the ambulance. Once in the ambulance, patient can be kept covered and warm with blankets and sheets.
- High probability that a large number of self-evacuated patients will flood the hospital campus.
- Hospitals should plan to prevent patient flooding, have a decontamination facility, and further manage patients from a SCMCI.

M. Lynn
University of Miami Miller School of Medicine, Jackson Memorial Hospital, Department of Surgery, Miami, FL, USA
e-mail: mlynn@med.miami.edu

© Springer Nature Switzerland AG 2019
M. Lynn et al. (eds.), *Disasters and Mass Casualty Incidents*,
https://doi.org/10.1007/978-3-319-97361-6_14

Prevention of Patient Flooding

Hospital security guards/police, regardless of their number, will most certainly be insufficient to prevent hundreds, if not thousands of panicked self-evacuees from flooding into the hospital.

* The most likely solution is to construct a gated perimeter fence around the hospital.

Decontamination

* Large urban medical centers in the community should plan for a large decontamination facility to handle a few hundred contaminated patients.
* Criteria to construct a decontamination facility (Fig. 14.1):
  – Preferably in open air.
  – If in closed spaces (cities with severe winter), assure adequate ventilation.
  – Available water source.
  – Contaminated water should drain into the city sewage system, not into the rain collection system.

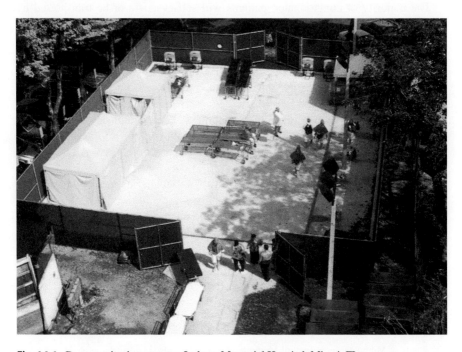

Fig. 14.1 Decontamination area at a Jackson Memorial Hospital, Miami, FL

- If no sewage system is available, an underground container, to collect contaminated water, may be a good alternative.
- Arrival and departure of ambulances to and from the decontamination facility should be one way. NO U-TURNS.
- The decontamination facility should be divided into two separate areas, with a clear boundary separating them:
  - Contaminated (HOT)
  - Clean

Planning of the Contaminated Area

- Decontamination team (must wear protective gear):
  - Team leader
  - Anesthesiologists/nurse anesthetists
  - Triage officer
  - Decontaminators
  - Emergency department (ED) physicians
  - Nurses
  - Respiratory therapists
  - Transporters (escorts)
  - Security guards
- Intubation corner for patients arriving in respiratory failure:
  - Standard intubation equipment and medications
- Chemical cart – with standard medications and antidotes for common chemical agents.
- Distinct showers for ambulatory and nonambulatory patients should be available in the contaminated area.
- "Fenced" stretchers should be available, to allow the contaminated water to drain off the stretcher (Fig. 14.2).
- Planning for the clean area:
  - Personnel (Does not need to wear protective gear):
    - Team leader
    - Triage officer
    - ED physicians
    - Nurses
    - Respiratory therapists
    - Transporters (escorts)
  - Chemical cart – with standard medications and antidotes for common chemical agents.
  - Clean stretchers and wheelchairs should be available to which patients will be transferred after decontamination.
  - Colored charts, by severity (severe-red, moderate-yellow, mild-green), with temporary medical record numbers and matching wristbands.

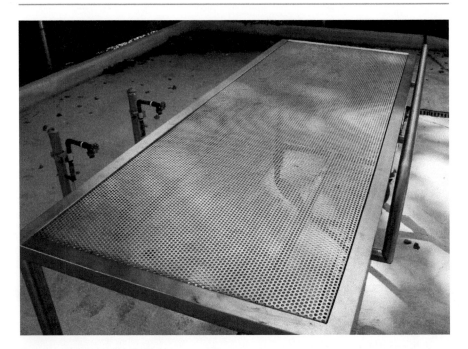

Fig. 14.2 "Fenced" stretcher

Flow of Patients (Fig. 14.3)

- Arrival of contaminated patient at entrance of decontamination facility.
- Triage between ambulatory and nonambulatory.
- All patients are undressed, receive a prenumbered wristband, and their clothing is tagged with the same number, for future identification.
- Nonambulatory patients are triaged between normal and abnormal respirations.
- Patients with abnormal respirations are diverted to the intubation corner.
    Note: Patients with respiratory failure should be intubated prior to decontamination.
- Ambulatory and nonambulatory patients are decontaminated at their respective areas.
- After decontamination, patients may walk or be transported to the clean area.
- At the clean area, patients are triaged according to the severity of contamination.
- Comatose patients and infants are photographed to facilitate later identification.
- Patients receive the colored chart according to their severity and with the same number as the wristband.
- Patients receive medications and antidotes as medically indicated.
- Minimal documentation is performed at the clean site: severity of the patient and medications received.
- Patients are transported to the respective in-hospital treatment site, according to severity.

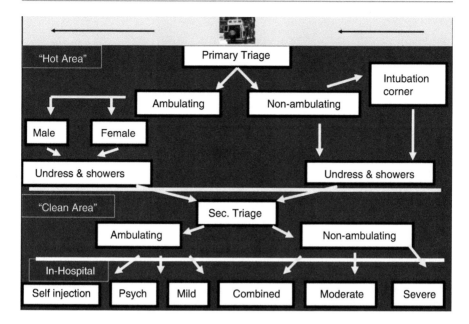

Fig. 14.3 Patient flow at the decontamination area

In-Hospital Treatment Sites

- Severe/moderate (nonambulatory):
  - Patients who need ventilatory support and/or hemodynamically unstable
  - Physicians, one of whom is a team leader
  - Nurses
  - Clerks
  - Transporters/escorts
  - Equipment:
    - Ventilators
    - Oxygen and suction
    - Monitors
    - Standard disposable ICU equipment
    - Medications/antidotes
    - Protocols based on symptoms
- Moderate/mild (ambulatory):
  - All ambulatory patients
  - Physicians, one of whom is a team leader
  - Nurses
  - Clerks
  - Transporters/escorts:
    - Oxygen, suction
    - Monitors
    - Standard medical ED equipment
    - Medications/antidotes and protocols based on symptoms

Medical Principles for the Management of a "Dirty Bomb"

15

Mauricio Lynn

Definition

"Dirty bomb" is an explosive device (ex: TNT) with the addition of radioactive material.

It is also named radiation dispersal device (RDD).

Medical Management

Since patients will suffer conventional injuries after an explosion, the presence of radioactive debris may not be diagnosed until the patient is assessed with a radiation spectrometer.

Therefore, the presence of radioactivity needs to be suspected after any explosion related to terrorism or any explosion at a location that uses or stores radioactive materials.

The medical priorities are the management of conventional injuries and should follow the principles of the Advanced Trauma Life Support (ATLS) ®.

Decontamination of these patients may be performed before during or after the resuscitation and stabilization of conventional injuries.

M. Lynn
University of Miami Miller School of Medicine, Jackson Memorial Hospital,
Department of Surgery, Miami, FL, USA
e-mail: mlynn@med.miami.edu

© Springer Nature Switzerland AG 2019
M. Lynn et al. (eds.), *Disasters and Mass Casualty Incidents*,
https://doi.org/10.1007/978-3-319-97361-6_15

Emergency Department Preparedness for "Dirty Bomb"

When planning the specific response for a "dirty bomb," in addition to the conventional planning, an emergency department (ED)/trauma center (TC – if applicable) should have large quantities of plastic rolls in storage that will be used to cover and protect equipment from contamination.

When the notification is received of an explosion with the potential for radioactive debris, the ED/TC must activate the hospital plan for a conventional event and follow the pertinent checklist, as described previously.

In addition, the ED/TC should do the following:
- Cover the floor, stretchers, wheelchairs, beds, and carts with the plastic rolls.
- Assess the patient at the triage area, including the use of a radiation spectrometer or other radiation detection devices.
- If patient is contaminated but otherwise stable from a trauma perspective, perform decontamination.
- If the patient is contaminated but in critical condition, stabilize the patient following ATLS® guidelines, including emergency surgery if needed. Perform decontamination once the patient is stable.
- When the event is over, discard the plastic covers, wash the ED/TC, and check for retained contamination.

Part III

Special Considerations in Management of Sudden Mass Casualty Incidents

Maritime Sudden Mass Casualty Incidents

16

Mauricio Lynn

Introduction

On a cruise ship, there is an average of two physicians and three nurses on call for emergencies 24 h a day. Both the doctors and nurses are emergency medicine specialists.

There is an average of one ventilator, 3–4 cardiac monitors, 5–8 pulse oxymeters, and one infirmary bed per 1000 passengers. Most of the ships do not have an operating room.

Each infirmary has the capability to provide critical care to one patient for 3–5 days.

It is possible that among the passengers, there will be a surgeon(s), anesthesiologist(s), trauma/critical care nurses, or other specialized medical personnel.

If we use the definition that a sudden mass casualty incident (SMCI) is a "temporary state of insufficiency" (lack of enough personnel, equipment, supplies, evacuation) as described previously, every incident aboard a cruise ship (e.g., explosion) that exceeds one severely injured patient may be considered a SMCI.

Assumptions

The management of a SMCI on a passenger ship at sea assumes the following conditions:
- The cruise line/ship has a plan to respond to a SMCI.
- The plan should include the following:
  - The ship's *surge capacity* scheme for staff, space, supplies, beds (stretchers)

M. Lynn
University of Miami Miller School of Medicine, Jackson Memorial Hospital,
Department of Surgery, Miami, FL, USA
e-mail: mlynn@med.miami.edu

© Springer Nature Switzerland AG 2019
M. Lynn et al. (eds.), *Disasters and Mass Casualty Incidents*,
https://doi.org/10.1007/978-3-319-97361-6_16

- Method to call for passengers who are medical professionals and are willing to help
- Predetermined alternate spaces onboard the ship that will be used to provide medical care if the number of patients exceeds the infirmary's capacity
- Mechanism for the deployment of extra equipment such as stretchers and supplies to predetermined alternate treatment areas
– Evacuation considerations:
  - Medical condition of the patient(s) and urgency for evacuation
  - Existence of a helipad onboard the ship
  - Availability of rescue/medical helicopters in the area
  - Distance to the closest port-of-call
  - Medical capabilities at the closest port-of-call
– Medical care
  - Remember, the majority of patients in a SMCI aboard a ship will be walking wounded.
  - Medical care should follow Advance Trauma Life Support (ATLS) ® principles.
  - Tourniquets may need to be used for limb hemorrhage. Caution needs to be used when applying improvised tourniquets, as they may worsen the bleeding!
  - Priorities for evacuation need to be established after patients are treated and stabilized.

Telemedicine to Manage Sudden Mass Casualty Incidents Remotely

17

Mauricio Lynn

Introduction

Telemedicine is gaining increasing popularity in recent years as a new approach to assist with patient care in remote locations, where expert physicians may not be available. Today, most medical personnel have cellular phones with cameras capable of transmitting still images and videos to experts all around the world. For these reasons, some advocate the use of telemedicine to manage disasters in remote locations.

Assumptions

A few technological components need to be in place, both at the *sender and recipient* sites, for telemedicine to be practical:
- Cameras and screens.
- Network system: cable, wireless, or satellite internet.

The practical definitions and the differences between the medical response for planned mass gatherings or progressive disasters and sudden mass casualty incidents (SMCIs) were previously discussed.

There is little debate that telemedicine should be part of the response for a planned mass gathering such a large sporting event or concert and for a progressive epidemic. In this situation, there is time for all technological components to be in place and to troubleshoot unexpected system failures, before the beginning of the event or during its slow progression. Even for large hurricanes that may destroy

M. Lynn
University of Miami Miller School of Medicine, Jackson Memorial Hospital,
Department of Surgery, Miami, FL, USA
e-mail: mlynn@med.miami.edu

© Springer Nature Switzerland AG 2019
M. Lynn et al. (eds.), *Disasters and Mass Casualty Incidents*,
https://doi.org/10.1007/978-3-319-97361-6_17

telecommunications, there is enough time before landfall occurs to prepare a backup plan based on satellite communications.

Nevertheless, the use of telemedicine for SMCIs is questionable at best. Earthquakes, tsunamis with major flooding, tornados, and large-scale explosions may partially or completely destroy the communications infrastructure in the area, including at hospitals. Even when the foundation is intact, cellular signals and wireless Internet need to be available around the clock, at the scene, in the ambulances and at the hospitals, for telemedicine to be used without interruptions. This is usually not the case, and it is the reason why telemedicine should NOT be included in the standard response plan for SMCIs.

The only way for telemedicine to be practical in SMCIs is if all components of the response plan, such as first responders, ambulances, and hospitals have a backup plan based on satellite communications, which incurs prohibitive costs.

Challenges with Deceased and Body Parts Identification

18

Mauricio Lynn

Large-scale explosions and plane crashes are good models for sudden mass casualty incidents (SMCIs) and may cause a large number of deaths and dismembered or fragmented bodies.

The identification process of deceased and body parts in such situations is one of the greatest challenges of managing SMCIs (Fig. 18.1).

Below is the list of techniques and frequency of their use in identifying corpses and body parts after explosions:

- Personal recognition – 43%
- Fingerprinting – 19%
- Teeth examination – 13%

Fig. 18.1 Challenges in body parts identification after explosions

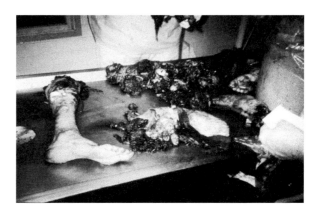

M. Lynn
University of Miami Miller School of Medicine, Jackson Memorial Hospital,
Department of Surgery, Miami, FL, USA
e-mail: mlynn@med.miami.edu

© Springer Nature Switzerland AG 2019
M. Lynn et al. (eds.), *Disasters and Mass Casualty Incidents*,
https://doi.org/10.1007/978-3-319-97361-6_18

- Personal documents – 10%
- DNA testing – 10%
- Specific signs – 5%

In rare situations, repatriation of deceased is necessary. It is important to remember that most countries prohibit air transport of bodies without previous embalmment.

Planning Exercises and Drills for Sudden Mass Casualty Incidents

19

Mauricio Lynn

Key components for planning exercises and drills for sudden mass casualty incidents (SMCIs):
- A plan for response to a SMCI needs to be written before the drill.
- Provide lectures to explain the plan to all individuals who may be involved in the response:
  - For pre-hospital: all first responders
  - For hospital: all medical, support personnel and administrators
- Organize tabletop exercises: Designed to bring together, into one room, all "players" that will respond to a SMCI (police, fire, EMS, hospitals, incident command, regional emergency operations center (REOC)). A large-scale incident is presented to them, and they have to resolve all challenges and pitfalls that it presents.
- Conduct sectorial *pre-hospital* exercises (Fig. 19.1): Constructed to train portions of the pre-hospital response separately. Examples:
  - Scene deployment to a SMCI and triage of patients: could be performed at the ambulance station parking lot, using inflatable dummies or cards with description of injuries.
  - Interaction between various ambulances and incident control: could be performed at an empty stadium parking lot, using inflatable dummies, where a few ambulances are deployed simultaneously. All paramedics perform triage, and the scene commander decides on transport priorities.
- Conduct sectorial *hospital* exercises: Constructed to train portions of the hospital response separately. Examples:
  - Deployment of triage, patient arrival and photography
  - Routes for emptying the emergency department

M. Lynn
University of Miami Miller School of Medicine, Jackson Memorial Hospital,
Department of Surgery, Miami, FL, USA
e-mail: mlynn@med.miami.edu

© Springer Nature Switzerland AG 2019
M. Lynn et al. (eds.), *Disasters and Mass Casualty Incidents*,
https://doi.org/10.1007/978-3-319-97361-6_19

  – Routes for influx of patients
  – Deployment of alternate care sites
• Deploy a full exercise, preferably with pre-hospital and hospital training together
  (Fig. 19.2).
• There is no substitute for a well-organized, full-scale exercise testing all compo-
  nents of the response simultaneously.

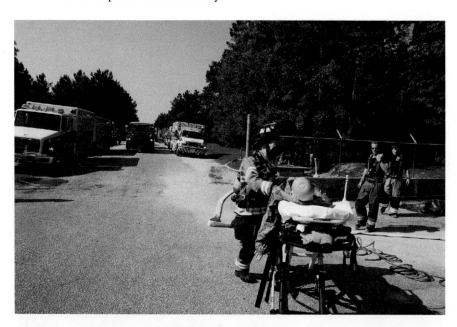

Fig. 19.1 Pre-hospital decontamination exercise

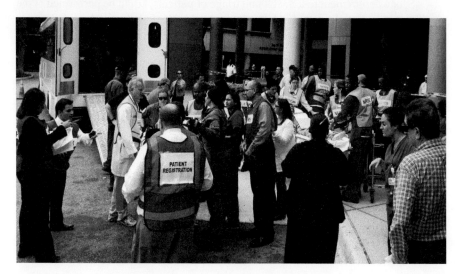

Fig. 19.2 Full hospital exercise conducted yearly at Jackson Memorial Hospital, Miami,
FL. Important issues to consider when organizing a SMCI drill

Pre-hospital

- First, there needs to be a detailed response plan for a SMCI.
- The drill needs to coincide to the written response plan.
- Try to make it a surprise.
- All agencies that are planned to be involved in a real SMCI should drill together:
  - Emergency medical services (EMS)
  - Fire department
  - Police
  - Regional emergency operations center (REOC)
- Test everything and focus on the common problematic areas:
  - Opening access routes to the scene of the SMCI, together with the local police
  - Setup of decontamination capability, when exercising the response to a chemical exposure
  - Evacuation routes from the scene to local hospital
  - Communications:
    - Among all participating ambulance services
    - Between ambulances, fire trucks, police and REOC
    - With local hospitals
- Use other cities/counties that are planned to exercise in the near future to critique the drill
- Modify the plan according to the lessons learned and repeat the drill to correct deficiencies
- Remember: A good, well-organized and expensive drill is cheaper than a bad drill.

Hospital

- First, there needs to be a detailed hospital response plan for a SMCI.
- The drill needs to coincide to the written response plan.
- Try to make it a surprise.
- All personnel planned to be involved in a real SMCI should drill together:
  - Hospital administrators
  - Abbreviated incident command
  - Medical and support personnel
- Test everything and focus on the common problematic areas:
  - Activation of security
  - Setting up the triage area
  - Emptying the emergency department (ED)
  - Deployment of equipment to alternate treatment sites
  - Control and deployment of extra personnel to treatment sites

- – Arrival of ambulances at triage area:
  - • One-way route
  - • NO U-turns
- – Transfer of patients from ambulance to hospital stretchers at the triage area, not in the ED
- – Identification of comatose and infant patients – photography
- – Registration of patients
- – Clinical management and control of patient destination
- – Activation of operating rooms, intensive care units, blood bank, radiology, laboratory and mental health
- – Activation of family/friends information center
- – Activation of media center
- – Incident command (IC)
- – Communications:
  - • With EMS
  - • Between treatment sites
  - • With IC
  - • With REOC
- • Use other hospitals that are planned to exercise in the near future to critique the drill.
- • Modify the plan according to the lessons learned and repeat the drill to correct deficiencies.
- • Remember: A good, well-organized and expensive drill is cheaper than a bad drill.

Deployment of Field Hospitals to Sudden Onset Disasters

20

Mauricio Lynn

Introduction

National or International deployments of field hospitals to sudden onset disasters (SOD), such as natural disasters, may be necessary when the event occurs in remote areas, with scarce medical support or when the local medical facilities are overwhelmed, destroyed, or damaged.

In most instances, a field hospital will temporarily replace the local medical facility and provide emergency medical and surgical care to the general population. Because the deployment of a field hospital may be several hours after the incident occurred, it is unlikely to have to treat a large number of critical patients directly related to the SOD.

Field hospitals need to be deployed by organizations that are completely self-sufficient with respect to personnel, equipment, and air assets and that perform training and exercises on a consistent basis. Military field hospitals should be considered the gold standard.

This chapter will describe the most important issues to consider when planning deployment of a field hospital.

Information Gathering

- Immediately after a large-scale SOD occurred, with the potential to deploy a field hospital, the *major news networks* should be used to collect preliminary information about the magnitude of the destruction and the potential for a field hospital deployment. Early estimations of the number of casualties are usually inaccurate.

M. Lynn
University of Miami Miller School of Medicine, Jackson Memorial Hospital,
Department of Surgery, Miami, FL, USA
e-mail: mlynn@med.miami.edu

© Springer Nature Switzerland AG 2019
M. Lynn et al. (eds.), *Disasters and Mass Casualty Incidents*,
https://doi.org/10.1007/978-3-319-97361-6_20

Pioneer Team

- After the decision to deploy a field hospital has been made by the government, a small pioneer team should be deployed to the area.
- The composition of the pioneer team should be as follows:
  - Team commander
  - Medical advisor
  - Logistics advisor
  - Search and Rescue advisor
  - Security officer
- The mission of the pioneer team:
  - Assess the area of the SOD, preferably by air
  - Learn the magnitude of destruction of the medical facilities (if applicable) and the major medical needs
  - Evaluate the need for search and rescue teams
  - Notify the field hospital commander regarding the findings
  - Recommend the final size and constitution of the field hospital
  - Decide the location of the field hospital (see below)
- After the final decision to deploy is made, the members of the pioneer team should decide where to place the field hospital. Criteria to choose the location:
  - Grounds next/close to the damaged medical facility, if possible.
  - The grounds should have good water drainage, to prevent flooding of tents in rainy seasons.
  - Do not use buildings because of safety considerations (thousands of after-shocks after a major earthquake).
  - The location of the field hospital could be easily secured (gated facilities, stadiums).
  - There should be enough space next to the field hospital to open a landing zone (LZ), for supplies and evacuation of patients.
  - Pioneer team should have satellite communications since cellular towers may be destroyed after a major earthquake.
- *Security*
  - There is a need for robust security for every deployment of personnel to remote disaster areas, whether it is a national or international mission (Fig. 20.1).

Logistically Self-Sufficient

- The field hospital needs to be logistically self-sufficient in the following areas, considering air transport limitations:
- Electricity (generators).
- Lodging (tents).
- Do not use or purchase local water (Fig. 20.2).
- Safe food should be flown in with the logistics.

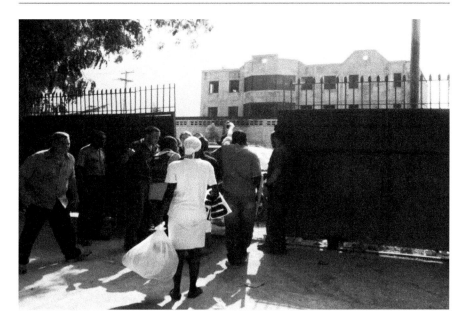

Fig. 20.1 Robust security at the entrance of an Israeli field hospital in Haiti, 2010

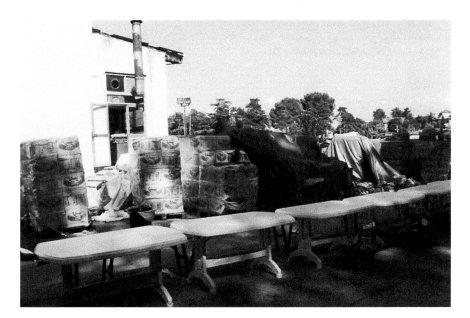

Fig. 20.2 Large quantities of water at an Israeli field hospital in Adapazarı, Turkey, 1998

- Showers and toilets.
- Heavy lifting machinery such as forklifts.
- Large number of vehicles/ambulances (if applicable) for patient transport and for
  the transportation of field hospital managers to city meetings and other missions.

Public Health

- Onset of a viral/bacterial gastrointestinal outbreak could be harmful for the personnel and significantly impair their mission.
- It is imperative to institute strict discipline with respect to public health, following the rules below:
  - Hand washing.
  - Use of alcohol-based hand hygiene products.
  - Patients and personnel should have separate toilets.
  - Do not use local water for drinking or showering.
  - Only verified food should be ingested.
  - Daily toilet cleaning.

Interaction for Local Authorities

- It is important to realize that the field hospital is a "visitor."
- The mayor/commissioner/representative is the incident commander (IC) at the affected city/area.
- It is the responsibility of the IC to decide the location of all field hospitals when there are more than one deployed.

Collaboration with Other Teams

- In the aftermath of a major SOD such as earthquakes, it is common to have many deployed field hospitals from all over the world.
- Not all field hospitals have the same capacity and capability to provide specialized medical care.
- It is important for the IC of the affected city/area to meet with representatives from all the field hospitals and perform an audit of their medical specialties, as this will prevent duplication.
- A citywide triage criteria and transport destinations should be set at this meeting, according to patient's condition and medical needs.

Complete Hospital

- The population in the city/area after a natural disaster may experience acute medical or surgical conditions.
- By default, patients will arrive at the local medical facility that has been damaged or destroyed.
- Patients should then be redirected to the field hospital deployed next to the local medical facility.

- Common medical/surgical conditions:
  - Surgical emergencies
  - Traumatic emergencies, related or not to the SOD
  - Increased number of deliveries
  - Penetrating eye injuries
  - Acute coronary syndromes
  - Acute exacerbation of asthma
- Suggested medical specialties to be deployed in the aftermath of a SMCI, most commonly earthquakes, hurricanes, or floods:
  - General surgery/trauma/burns
  - Orthopedics
  - Obstetrics
  - Ophthalmology
  - General anesthesia
  - Neonatology/pediatrics
  - Medicine: cardiology/pulmonary
  - Critical care
- It is important to have all specialties in place once the field hospital announces its opening. It prevents patients from walking from one field hospital to another to find appropriate medical care.

Adjacent Landing Zone (LZ)

- When choosing the location, it is important to keep in mind the need to have a LZ in proximity to the field hospital.
- The LZ may later be used for flying in medical supplies, logistics, humanitarian supplies (food, water), and evacuation of patients to hospitals outside the disaster area.

Central Triage and Evacuation for the Affected City/Area
(Fig. 20.3)

- Critical patients should be evacuated by air (if applicable) to hospitals outside the affected city/area, where optimal medical care can be provided.
- Not all field hospitals in the affected city/area will have an adjacent LZ.
- It is therefore important for the IC of the disaster to designate one or more "central triage and evacuation" places where patients could be transported by ground. Patients should be triaged according to severity and air evacuated to hospitals outside the disaster zone.
- The "central triage and evacuation" should be in a secured area, large enough to include medical tents for triage and landing capability for helicopters. An open stadium is an ideal place.

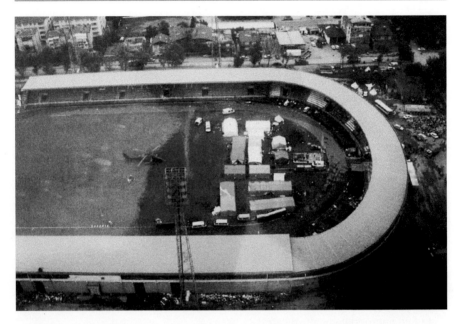

Fig. 20.3 Central triage and evacuation in the city of Duzce, Turkey, 1998

Media Management

- Every deployment planning should include the protocols to handle the media. A few suggestions:
    - Plan a distinct area/tent in the "campus" of the field hospital for media deployment
    - Appoint a spokesman. He/she will be the only contact with the media during the deployment period. In the USA, this is the responsibility of the public information officer
    - Schedule frequent media debriefings, at least twice daily

After observing a wide variation in medical aid capacities, competencies, and adherence to professional ethics in various disasters, the WHO has published classification and minimum standards for foreign medical teams (FMT) in SOD.

This document sets the minimum requirements that a field hospital must have to be able to provide proper medical aid in disaster areas.

Hospital Security Considerations During Sudden Mass Casualty Incidents

21

Henry Morgenstern

Hospitals are meant to be, above all, safe places. Nevertheless, attempts to attack hospitals by suicide bombers in Israel and active shooter events at hospitals in the USA (Lebanon Hospital, Bronx, NY) have put security back at the top of hospital planning agendas.

Testing and improving hospital security should be part of a mature MCI plan. Normal access control to the hospital may be unmanageable due to sudden surge.

Some suggestions that may help improve the hospital security plan are discussed next.

Risk and Threat Assessment

According to the FBI, incidents of mass shooting have increased 20-fold since 2000. In view of the startling increase in violent incidents, it is recommended to perform frequent assessments of the risks and threats and consequently modify the hospital security plan accordingly.

Access of Ambulances and Triage Area

- Hospital security staff should have basic training in behavioral recognition so that they can scan arrivals and be vigilant for personnel with suspicious activity.
- Concentrate security staff at the most volatile point which is the *triage area* where most ambulances arrive.
- Arriving ambulances should be inspected to be certain they are transporting patients.

H. Morgenstern
Security Solutions International INC, Miami, FL, USA
e-mail: contact@homelandsecurityssi.com

© Springer Nature Switzerland AG 2019
M. Lynn et al. (eds.), *Disasters and Mass Casualty Incidents*,
https://doi.org/10.1007/978-3-319-97361-6_21

- Families and friends should be directed to the family/friends information center and asked for basic identification before entering the hospital.

Parking

- Vehicles may pose another threat. Therefore, security staff at entrances of parking garages should inspect arriving vehicles and ask for basic identification.

Hospital Lockdown

- Some events, such as mass chemical contamination (Sarin Gas Attack, Tokyo), may require hospital lockdown to prevent contaminated patients entering the hospital at other entrances apart from the main triage and admitting area.

Communications

- As discussed previously, security personnel should have portable two-way radios, on a different frequency than the medical one.

Exercises

Recommended topics for security exercises and drills:
- Behavioral recognition of suspicious activity
- Vehicle inspection at entrance of parking garages
- Hospital lockdown:
  - Active shooter
  - Prevention of patient flooding
- Triage area security:
  - Media control
  - Ambulance inspection
  - Influx of patients
- Control and direction of families and friends

Ethical Considerations in Sudden Mass Casualty Incidents and Disasters

22

Alex Canales

Introduction

Sudden mass casualty incidents (SMCIs) and disasters may overwhelm the local and regional healthcare systems, and it will be more evident in events where the infrastructure of the city is partially or completely destroyed, such as in earthquakes, hurricanes, and devastating flooding.

In addition, evacuation and transport capabilities of patients outside the disaster area may be compromised, therefore making the problem even worst.

There will be times when major ethical decisions will need to be made with respect to patient outcome, more often in scenarios in which the risks to medical staff are higher than the benefits of continuing futile medical care.

Each hospital needs to have an ethical committee, permanent or ad hoc, to assist medical personnel with these difficult resolutions.

Below are scenarios and medical conditions that require challenging decision making.

When Is the Hospital and/or Region Overwhelmed?

Scenarios may be cataloged into levels 0–4 with respect to amount of resources needed to handle SMCIs and disasters.

A. Canales
Jackson Memorial Hospital, Miami Beach, FL, USA
e-mail: alexander.canales@jhsmiami.org

© Springer Nature Switzerland AG 2019
M. Lynn et al. (eds.), *Disasters and Mass Casualty Incidents*,
https://doi.org/10.1007/978-3-319-97361-6_22

Level 0

This is the default norm of an organized health-care system and is like a typical day in an emergency department. In general, there are no restrictions in resources, and optimal care is provided to all patients at this level.

Level 1

Transition to level 1 occurs when the capacity of a medical center, but not a medical region, is overwhelmed by a sudden patient surge resulting in temporary staff shortages (SMCI definition: temporary state of insufficiency, as discussed previously).

In this situation, the regional emergency operations center (REOC) is responsible to evenly distribute patients among area hospitals. Rarely, an institution may need to divert patients to other institutions, assuming it will not result in death, loss of function, or patient deterioration.

Level 2

Transition to level 2 occurs when the response required after a large-scale SMCI exceeds the medical region's capacity.

The goal is to save the maximum number of lives.
- First triage patients into three categories:
  - Most seriously injured (likely to die with treatment) – black tagged
  - Walking wounded (likely to live without treatment) – green tagged
  - Everyone else (likely to live with treatment or die without treatment) – red tagged
- Prioritize red-tagged patients who have conditions that are the most emergent and likely to survive

Level 3

Physical insults like earthquakes or epidemic illness can devastate a medical region's capacity. This scenario overwhelms the medical region's capacity for red-tagged patients.
- Must decide when it is acceptable to dismiss medical staff.
- Most likely, black-tagged patients will not be treated.
- Consider "firing" medical staff to ease the burden of guilt for patient abandonment.

- If possible, first insure that hospitals can
  - Assess all incoming patients
  - Monitor and attend to all red-tagged patients
  - Possess sufficient staff
  - Maintain functional infrastructure
  - Ensure cooperation of patients and their families
- Then optimize capacity:
  - Timely discharge of patients
  - Add beds
  - Assemble supplies for easy access
  - Summon supplementary health-care workers like volunteers, dentists, and veterinarians
  - Set up medical facilities outside of the hospitals
  - Utilize all available space
  - Increase security staff
  - Evacuate patients whenever possible

Level 4

Scenario likely caused by viral illness.
- All patients are black tagged.
- Four defining characteristics:
  - Extremely contagious
  - Very high mortality
  - Global
  - Untreatable
- May have a health-care system without health-care workers.
- Strategy to reduce casualties:
  - Minimize human-to-human contact (social distancing) for as long as possible
  - Utilize available resources and infrastructure for research into effective treatment

Most likely, major ethical decisions will need to be made at levels 3 and 4.

An example of a challenging scenario would be a partially destroyed hospital in the aftermath of an earthquake and ventilated patients in an intensive care unit at a high floor. Elevators are not functioning, stairs partially destroyed.

The question is what to do with these patients?

This will be the case to discuss patient outcome with the ethical committee.

Mass Fatality Management in Mass Casualty Incidents

23

Alon D. Schwartz

Sudden mass causality incidents (SMCI) and disasters may be associated with a mass fatality incident (MFI) sometimes exceeding local capacity. A scheme to manage mass number of deceased needs to be integrated within the overall disaster plan of the city and region (Fig. 23.1).

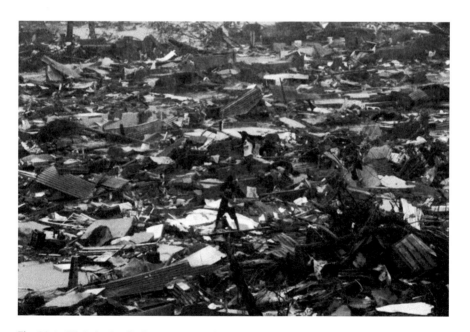

Fig. 23.1 High death toll after Typhoon Haiyan, Philippines, 2013

A. D. Schwartz
Trauma and Acute Care Surgery, Shaare Zedek Medical Center,
Department of General Surgery, Jerusalem, Israel
e-mail: alon.schwarz@jhsmiami.org

© Springer Nature Switzerland AG 2019
M. Lynn et al. (eds.), *Disasters and Mass Casualty Incidents*,
https://doi.org/10.1007/978-3-319-97361-6_23

The overall responsibility for body or remains identification is usually of the medical examiner office or the governmental pathology services of the region. Nevertheless, coordination with the police, fire department, and national health services is of key strategic importance.

Voluntary agencies may be involved with psychological support and pastoral care.

There are few principles that guide the multiple fatalities incident management:

- Provision of honest and accurate information at all times
- Avoidance of mistaken identity
- Respect for the deceased and the bereaved

Unlike routine casework, where human remains are processed at one station, a MFI remains are often processed in multiple stations due to the intensive work that is required. The data collection should be standardized and integrated to one central victim information center (VIC).

Identification

Several techniques may be used to identify the deceased, determine the cause of death, and return human remains to families:

- Digital media and photos
- Personal belongings
- Body and dental X-rays
- Finger prints
- Comparison between postmortem DNA specimens and DNA samples collected from the family

DNA may be obtained also from some personal effects bearing biological material. For that reason, a DNA specialist should be consulted before personal belongings are cleaned for photographing, cataloging, and returning to families.

Comprehensive X-rays documentation is made of appropriate cases to identify commingled remains, artifacts (jewelry, evidence, etc.) imbedded in human tissue, and evidence of antemortem skeletal injury, surgeries, or anomalies. Such features may aid in identification by correlation with antemortem medical records.

Human remains that lack typical identifying features (tissues without fingerprint, dental, or anthropological material) can often be identified through DNA. For this reason, morgue processing should include a station to obtain and preserve a specimen for DNA testing from each case processed.

Law enforcement may require that the remains be retained or partially retained for evidentiary purposes; thus, the morgue's storage capacity may need to be further enhanced.

Mass fatality disasters have the potential to be complicated with biological, chemical, or radiological agent exposure of the victims. In this case, body handling should include specialized assets to assist with decontamination of victims. Remains may need to be decontaminated before they are transported to the morgue. Because the setup for decontamination capability may not be immediately available, refrigerated storage of remains at the incident site may become necessary.

In certain disaster situations, there may not be remains to recover for identification, or the scientific efforts to establish identity fails. In situations like these, a legal authority may order a presumptive death certificate.

Data Distribution

Victim information center (VIC) should be established in conjunction with the management of a MIF. The objectives of a VIC are to collect and distribute data from and to families of victims. Interviewers should be limited to personnel specially trained in handling grieving individuals and may use standardized questionnaire forms. DNA collection from families can be performed with buccal swabs at this location. The center will also collect the reported missing person reports and will compare it with the data that is being collected.

Disposition

Traditional funeral practices include a variety of procedures designed to assist survivors of all religious practices and beliefs with the grieving process. Identification of the victim, however, is the first step in the process.

Government-ordered disposition by mass burial or cremation of unidentified victims creates numerous, and often unnecessary, complications for survivors. In addition to delay in completing the grieving process, survivors face challenges of settling legal affairs, determining rights of property ownership, and managing the welfare of the victim's offspring.

Both the World Health Organization (WHO) and the Pan American Health Organization (PAHO) advocate for identification of all disaster victims before final disposition, regardless of number of victims.

Epidemic Outbreak Myth

Review of past catastrophic disasters demonstrates that the risk of epidemic disease transmission from human remains is negligible. Unless the affected population was already experiencing a disease suitable for epidemic development, the catastrophic event cannot create such a situation. Most disaster victims die from traumatic events and not from preexisting disease.

Plan and Training

It will be imperative to ensure that the arrangements within plans are sufficiently realistic, resilient, and flexible to adapt to the unique challenges which will be encountered. When devising plans, training, and exercises, particular consideration should be given to the selection, support, and monitoring of those staff with roles which will expose them to situations in which they are dealing with victims and human remains, or with survivors, relatives, and friends of victims.

Part IV

Progressive and Slow Developing Disasters and Their Aftermath

Introduction

As discussed in the first section, the planning and response to sudden onset incidents should be different than the preparation for events that develop over a long period of time. This section focuses on the peculiar areas that need to be addressed when planning for progressive or slow onset disasters.

Shabnam Hafiz and Hahn Soe-Lin

Epidemiology of Injuries

Hurricanes and typhoons are slowly developing disaster scenarios, thus, allowing the population, prehospital emergency response systems, and hospitals to prepare prior to storm impact (Fig. 24.1).

A hurricane disaster passes through three distinct phases:

- Prearrival and preparation phase: 1–7 days prior to impact
- Hurricane impact phase: 12–48 hours
- Posthurricane rescue and recovery phase: 1–4 weeks

During the prearrival phase, injuries are related to evacuation and preparation activities. Falls from ladders during window shutter installation, interpersonal violence, and motor vehicle crash-related injuries are prevalent.

During the impact phase, the total number of trauma victims presenting to hospitals is actually lower, since people who did not evacuate shelter in place and EMS system suspend services due to road safety conditions. Nevertheless, several interpersonal violence cases, predominantly gunshot wounds, may occur. Therefore, maintaining full surgical capacity at trauma centers during the impact phase is still important.

Most hurricane-related injuries occur during the posthurricane rescue and recovery phase over a protracted period of time. Falls from height, power tool-related

S. Hafiz · H. Soe-Lin (✉)
Ryder Trauma Center, Jackson Memorial Hospital,
Department of Surgery, Miami, FL, USA
e-mail: Hahn.soelin@jhsmiami.org

© Springer Nature Switzerland AG 2019
M. Lynn et al. (eds.), *Disasters and Mass Casualty Incidents*,
https://doi.org/10.1007/978-3-319-97361-6_24

133

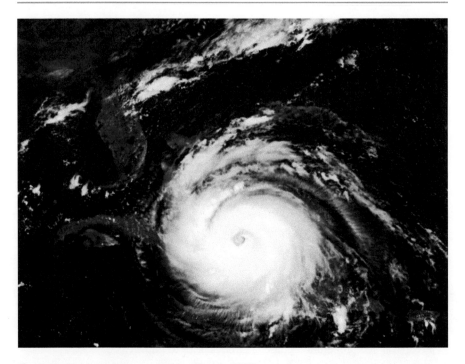

Fig. 24.1 Hurricane Irma approaching Florida, 2017

injuries, and interpersonal violence are common. A significant number of burn injuries due to propane camping stoves and grills used during posthurricane power outages occur as well. Frequently, a large number of medical patients and patients with
special medical needs such as hemodialysis and long-term ventilator dependence
present to emergency rooms and require significant hospital resources.

One third of patients with hurricane-related injuries require operative interventions with 49% orthopedic procedures, 34% trauma operations, and 19% other procedures, such as hand injuries.

Personnel and Hospital Planning

Personal planning for hospitals, in preparation for hurricanes, requires unique
staffing considerations. Essential medical and support personnel should be
grouped into team A, which remains on site during the impact phase and team B,
which will relieve team A in the immediate aftermath and as soon as local travel
is deemed safe.

It is advisable to assign staff to team A and team B in the beginning of each cal-
endar year or at the beginning of each hurricane season allowing long-term personal
planning for employees ahead of an actual hurricane. Hospital organizations should
consider accommodating family members and pets of the employees assigned to

team A since these families may not be able to evacuate the area and require a safe place to shelter during impact. Resources for these family members and team A should be allotted for several days, given that power outages, waste leaks, and downed electric lines may make egress impossible immediately postimpact.

Responsibilities for Team A Staff Members

- Continue care of current hospital inpatient population.
- Attend additional special needs patients such as hemodialysis patients and home ventilator dependent patients.
- Surgical trauma teams to address a moderate number of patients with
- immediate life-threatening injuries, such as gun violence and stab wounds.
- Elective operations and procedures are suspended to prepare for potential increase in hospital capacity.

Responsibilities of Team B Staff Members

- Surgical trauma teams to address significant number of injured patients in the immediate posthurricane period
- Medical care for the current inpatient population
- Gradual return to normal hospital operations

Hospital planning requires extensive preparation prior to hurricane season with focus on:
- Fuel supplies for backup power generators for several days to weeks, depending on local capacities
- Medical supplies to guarantee full hospital operations for 2–4 weeks
- Food supplies and drinking water for patients, staff, and families for at least 2 weeks

Recovery

The recovery phase includes:
- Assessment of damage to the hospital infrastructure and immediate repair of damage to critical infrastructure, compromising current hospital operations
- Close communication between regional incident command systems and hospital disaster incident command to coordinate medical needs for the community
- Assessment of the demand and capacity situation within the hospital system, and request for external help (e.g., FEMA) based on local situation
- Gradual return to normal operations with consideration to a protracted surge of trauma patients over several weeks, presenting with injuries related to recovery and reconstruction activities

Planning and Response for Biological Epidemics and Bioterrorism

Mauricio Lynn

Introduction

Information about specific treatment of anthrax, smallpox, botulinum, Ebola, and other infectious diseases can be found elsewhere.

The purpose of this chapter is to discuss the major challenges regarding community planning and response to the purposeful spread of a biological agent, most commonly known as bioterrorism.

Definition

The most common and acceptable definition of bioterrorism is the use of microorganisms or toxins to produce death or disease in humans, animals, or plants.

The final outcome of a biological epidemic may be thousands of people sick. Nevertheless, because of the slow evolution of an infectious agent, it is unlikely that one hospital will be overwhelmed with hundreds of a patient during the first day(s) of the event. Therefore, biological epidemics are classified as *progressive disasters*, as previously discussed.

The community and hospital disaster plan should reflect the unique characteristic of an infectious outbreak and focus on the response once it became obvious that a biological epidemic is under way. This is the major challenge when managing such an event.

M. Lynn
University of Miami Miller School of Medicine, Jackson Memorial Hospital, Department of Surgery, Miami, FL, USA
e-mail: mlynn@med.miami.edu

© Springer Nature Switzerland AG 2019
M. Lynn et al. (eds.), *Disasters and Mass Casualty Incidents*,
https://doi.org/10.1007/978-3-319-97361-6_25

Threat

Some countries may have the capabilities to weaponize biological agents due to several reasons:
- Equipment used to grow bacteria and viruses may be found at hospitals and industry.
- There is no need to store large stockpiles of the biological agent.
- It is extremely easy to hide from low enforcement authorities.
- Delivery systems, such as planes that spread pesticides, are already in use in agriculture. (Fig. 25.1)
- Most likely, the start of the event will be "silent."
- National or international transmission may be very rapid due to massive air travel.

Challenges

We will now describe four major challenges when managing a biological outbreak and offer possible solutions:
- As mentioned above, the *number one challenge* is to know if a biological attack actually started or it is just a bad flu season.
  - The most common initial signs of any biological agent will be flu-like symptoms, and patients will likely turn to their primary care physician or to emergency departments (EDs), depending on the severity of symptoms.
  - It will be up to the astute clinician to discern between common infectious diseases and rare or eradicated agents such anthrax, smallpox, or Ebola.

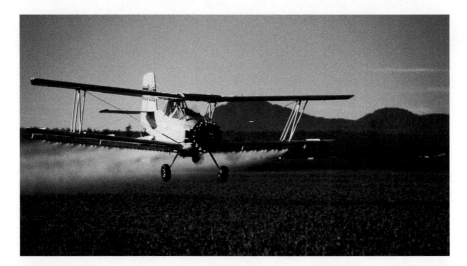

Fig. 25.1 Agriculture plane that may be used to spread a biological agent

- High index of suspicion and consultation with local public health authorities is crucial for the initial investigation and management.
- Another possible clue that a biological outbreak is under way is a higher incidence of patients with flu-like symptoms and fever outside the flu season. Local clinics and EDs need to report any unusual increase of sick patients to the local public health authorities.
- The *second* important challenge is to *prevent panic* among the local population.
  - Lack of knowledge regarding what to do is the most common cause of panic among people living in an area where a biological attack just happened.
  - It is the responsibility of the local public health authorities, together with the Center for Disease Control (CDC) to publish guidelines in the media and local clinics and direct the local population about what to do. Examples: "Stay home," "avoid gatherings," "evacuate," when to go to the ED, what is the treatment for the specific infection and where they can receive the antibiotics, whether for treatment or prophylaxis (see below).
- A community plan for antibiotics distribution needs to be in place in case that the infection requires specific treatment or prophylaxis.
  - Two important methods for antibiotics distribution are as follows:
    - Central distribution location(s) in the community: The down side of this method is the establishment of long lines and gathering of potentially infected with noninfected people.
    - Home-to-home distribution by community postman: This is probably a better distribution method since the residents stay home, reducing the risk of further spread of the infection.
- Preparing hospitals to receive a large number of infected people over a period of days, weeks, and even months may be the most difficult challenge to overcome.
  - Human-to-human transmission of some infectious epidemics, such as Ebola, occurs through direct contact and therefore requires isolation of the patient. Other infections, such as bubonic plague, may be transmitted through respiratory droplets and may require isolation in negative pressure rooms.
  - During a biological attack, the number of infected patients that may present to a single hospital is unpredictable. May range from a few dozens to hundreds and possibly thousands. Construction of hundreds of negative pressure rooms is financially prohibitive, considering the rarity of such events.
  - Therefore, every hospital needs to have basic planning in case a biological event occurs. The most cost-effective solution is to plan for a "designated isolation floor," usually the upper floor of the hospital, with access limited to infected patients and health-care providers dressed in protective gear. (Fig. 25.2)
  - If the number of infected patients exceeds the number of designated beds at all hospitals in the community, military field hospitals may need to be deployed at isolated areas of the city.

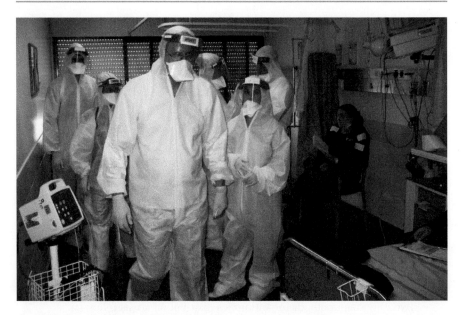

Fig. 25.2 Designated isolation floor during a biological drill at an Israeli hospital

Management of Late Effects of Radiological Incidents

26

Asaf Kedar

Radiological incidents refer to any incident, accidental or intentional, with exposure to radioactive material.

Known events are the accidents at the Chernobyl nuclear plant in Ukraine (1986) and the Fukushima nuclear accident in Japan (2011) (Fig. 26.1). However, an accident at a medical or industrial installation, or transportation of radioactive material, can lead to exposure of radioactive material and radiation injuries.

An intentional exposure, such as detonation of a "dirty bomb" (also known as radiation dispersal device – RDD), may produce combined blast injuries and radiation exposure.

Irradiation of human cells may result from direct exposure (whole/partial body), deposition, inhalation, and ingestion of food and water. This will lead to acute and delayed effects, which may involve every major organ system. Depending on the dose, acute changes may occur within minutes to days or weeks and may include injury to the skin, bone marrow, gastrointestinal tract, and neurovascular system. Chronic changes may take many months or years to become evident, and include the development of cutaneous ulcers, malignancies (e.g., thyroid cancer, leukemia, breast cancer, lung cancer), growth retardation in children, cataracts, infertility, and fetal abnormalities.

Therefore, the medical personnel involved in managing such events, on the short and long terms, will include:

- Trauma surgeons
- Emergency medicine physicians
- Radiation safety officers
- Radiation oncologists
- Nuclear medicine physicians

A. Kedar
Jackson Memorial Hospital, University of Miami Miller School of Medicine, DeWitt Daughtry Family Department of Surgery, Division of Trauma/Critical Care/Burns, Miami, FL, USA

© Springer Nature Switzerland AG 2019
M. Lynn et al. (eds.), *Disasters and Mass Casualty Incidents*,
https://doi.org/10.1007/978-3-319-97361-6_26

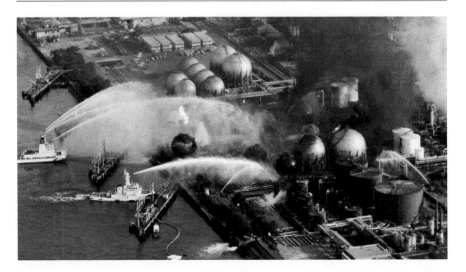

Fig. 26.1 Fukushima nuclear meltdown, Japan, 2011

- Hematologists
- Medical oncologists
- Infectious disease specialists
- Gastroenterologists

The clinical features of radiation and specific treatment may be found elsewhere. We will discuss the organizational aspects when managing radiation events.

The response to such incidents is complex and requires multiple agencies, good communication, organization, planning, education, protocols, and practice.

The overall response for a radiological incident is divided into three phases:

- *Early phase:* Lasts hours to days, begins with the incident (may be predicted in case of an accident with no leak initially but expected to happen within a few hours). This phase will include:
  - Guidance for sheltering or evacuations
  - Distribution of potassium iodide (KI) prophylactic treatment
  - Distribution of protective gear to limit exposure of rescue personal
- *Intermediate phase:* Lasts weeks to months. It begins after source and release are under control (not necessarily stopped, but no longer expanding). This phase includes:
  - Activities intended to reduce or avoid dose exposure to the public such as relocation, which is the principle of protective action against whole body external exposure.
  - Instruction for consuming food and drinking water.
  - Continuing to control and limit emergency worker exposure (total dose incurred over entire response).
  - Plan and control reentry.

- Prepare for late phase cleanup.
- This phase may overlap the early phase and late phase.
- *Late phase:* Lasts months to years. It begins when recovery actions are started and ends when all recovery actions have been completed.
  - This phase includes cleanup and waste disposal.

Institutes and organizations need to provide responders and decision makers with plans and protocols that address radiological incidents and to ensure appropriate education and training.

Protocols and training materials may be obtained from:
- International Commission on Radiological Protection (ICRP)
- National Council on Radiation Protection and Measurements (NCRP)
- International Atomic Energy Agency (IAEA)
- American Nuclear Society (ANS)
- Health Physics Society (HPS)

Detailed information on the risks of radiological emergency response and worker protection procedures can be found:
- FRMAC "Radiological Emergency Response Health and Safety Manual" (DOE 2012)
- NCRP's "Management of Terrorist Events Involving Radioactive Material, Report No. 138" (NCRP 2001)
- "Responding to a Radiological or Nuclear Terrorism Incident: A Guide for Decision Makers, Report No. 165" (NCRP 2010)

The institutional protocols/manual should include the following:
- All aspects of conventional events as described previously in this book
- Detailed reports on radiation risk, injury, and treatment
- Risk management decision-making
- Public communication guidelines and protocols
- Personal protective gear protocol
- Cleanup and waste disposal protocols
- Lists of federal, state, and local agencies involve in managing radiological events
- List of specialized personnel (radiation safety officers, radiation oncologists, nuclear medicine physicians, hematologists, medical oncologists) including contact information, function, and location in case of radiological emergency
- List of special equipment needed:
  - Geiger-Muller detectors
  - Dosimeters
  - Kits for dicentric chromosome assay
  - Protective gear
  - Contamination control
  - Storage location
  - Scheduled maintenance
  - Function to collect instrument and operate it in case of emergency

Principle of Medical management of radiological event:
- Any explosion should be screened for radiological event.
- Rescue personal should be aware in any industrial/medical facility accident to look for evidence of a radiological event.
- Follow all the principle of SMCI and checklists.
- The medical priorities are the management of conventional injuries and should follow the principles of the Advanced Trauma Life Support (ATLS)®.
- Triage: Decision if priority is medical treatment or decontamination. If the decision is to manage the traumatic injuries first, decontamination needs to be performed as soon as possible.
- In contaminated area, all personal should have protective gear and time of exposure limited, according to instructions from radiation protocols.
- Consider to manage contaminated patients at alternate sites, such as tents, instead of emergency department.
- Contaminated areas should be well marked and have restricted access.
- Clinicians should communicate with radiation experts about their needs in simple and accurate terms, without abbreviations or unimportant information. Likewise, radiation experts should avoid technical jargon when addressing clinicians or administrators.
- Stockpile equipment and instruments:
  - Plastic rolls, used to cover stretchers, floors, and protect equipment.
  - Protective gear.
  - Potassium iodide.
  - Direction signs and marking of contaminated areas/instruments.
  - Radiological disposable bags, basins, sponges, and soap (for decontamination).
  - Identification vests, by function, are especially important when having protective clothing since everyone looks the same and makes it very difficult to identify the different functions and professions.
- Exercises and drills for radiological events.

Chronic Illnesses and Nutritional Support in the Aftermath of Disasters

27

Caleb J. Mentzer and D. Dante Yeh

When managing patients requiring both acute and chronic nutritional support, several topics need to be considered:
- Acute nutritional support of the healthy is not an emergency, but management of fluids and hydration may become one.
- Patients receiving chronic nutritional support will likely be unsupported for periods of time, depending upon their individual preparation and the support and planning of the home health providers. Health care providers will need to assess the urgent versus emergent needs of these individuals.
- Patient evacuation plans dictate ability to meet nutritional support needs.
- Support of chronic patients requires preplanning and institutional support. Shelters, hospitals, government organizations may be able to provide a range of services, from minimal to full support.
- The expiration time for parenteral nutrition (PN) solution is limited. However, expiration time for enteric feeds may be extended.
- Despite availability of nutritional support, significant loss of infrastructure (e.g., access to gasoline, lack of navigable roads) may delay delivery of support.

C. J. Mentzer (✉)
Memorial Hermann Hospital, Department of Surgery,
Division of Acute Care Surgery, University of Texas Health Science Center,
Houston, TX, USA

D. D. Yeh
Ryder Trauma Center, Department of Surgery, Miami, FL, USA

© Springer Nature Switzerland AG 2019
M. Lynn et al. (eds.), *Disasters and Mass Casualty Incidents*,
https://doi.org/10.1007/978-3-319-97361-6_27

Patient Factors in Nutritional Support

The delivery of nutritional support in the time of disasters is at times a patient-dependent process.
- Media hyperbole and patient apathy present conflicting outlook for patients.
- Ever-changing weather forecasts, with inaccurate predictions, may result in patients delaying evacuation, deciding to shelter in place, or last-minute evacuations.
- Only approximately 50% of patients will evacuate.
- Not all patients are "teachable" to care for themselves.

Institutional assistance for the nutritional support-dependent patient will be varied:
- *Evacuation out of disaster area:*
  - Evacuated patients are required to inform home health supply company of new location to arrange for delivery of nutritional support.
  - Some companies may not have service coverage to new location.
- *Shelter-in-place:*
  - Limited support will be available.
  - Pre-event planning with home health may preemptively supply the patient with required support.
- *Red Cross shelter* is a regular shelter with no medical support.
- *"Special needs" shelters:*
  - Limited space is available.
  - Preregistration is required.
  - Requires documentation of medical need.
  - Medical care is limited other than basic care and ability to transport to regional medical facilities.
  - May have volunteer nurses and physicians.
  - Required to have a generator and refrigeration, but patients must provide their own care.
  - Only 10–20% of patients elect this option.
- *Skilled nursing facilities:* these centers are under no obligation to accept patients and often have scarce resources.
- *Hospital admissions* during events are triaged.
  - Level 1 (highest acuity) through Level 8 (lowest acuity) based on acuity of therapy:
    - 85% of elective admissions are for infections of anti-infective agents.
    - 15% are for PN and cardiovascular infusion (e.g., inotropes).
  - Pain management (hospice and nonhospice)
    - Level 2.
    - Elective hospital admission is strongly encouraged.

Pharmacy Considerations

- Pharmacies must plan to ramp up production in the days leading up to disaster (e.g., blizzard, hurricane).
  - "Mandatory overtime": every pharmacist comes, to compound drugs and get them out of the pharmacy as quickly as possible.

Delivery of Nutritional Support

With limited resources, preplanning and improvised delivery of nutritional support is required. Duration of enteral and parenteral solutions varies.
- Nutrition is NOT an emergency.
- Maintaining fluid balance and *hydration status* is potentially life threatening.
- Options for hydration include *World Health Organization (WHO) Oral Rehydration Solutions (ORT)* and hypodermoclysis (i.e., subcutaneous injections).
- 3-in-1 (carbohydrates, amino acids, lipids) parenteral solutions have a stability of 8–9 days.
- 2-in-1 (carbohydrates, amino acids) parenteral solutions have a stability of 8 days.
- Duration of use before "expiration" is dictated by local boards of pharmacy.
- If no sedimentation is visible, one may consider using an "expired" parenteral solution if no other option is available, and the situation is dire.
- Enteral formulas have longer shelf life, but systems require changing tubes and reservoirs as frequently as every 24–48 h, due to infectious concerns.
- Some patients may be taught to deliver TPN without a home pump if a "programmable" drip set is available.

Recent Lessons Learned from Hurricanes Harvey and Irma
(Fig. 27.1)

- Getting gasoline was the #1 problem after the hurricane.
- Lack of infrastructural support (open roads, access to fuel, access to high water vehicles) remains a limiting factor in delivery of nutritional support to patients sheltered at home.
- Availability of pharmacy staff to prepare parenteral solutions was limited both in hospital and in outpatient setting.
- Loss of power, loss of auxiliary power sources, and flooded storages resulted in loss of stockpiled product.
- Generator support of pharmacy is critical, so existing stock is not lost after the disaster is over.

- Regional resources, from outside of disaster, were able to be reallocated to affected areas to address lack of supply.
- Plan for triage of supplies between branches.
- Development of "disaster nutritional support kit" (Fig. 27.2).

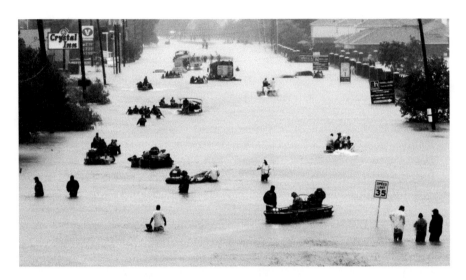

Fig. 27.1 City of Houston flooded after Hurricane Harvey, 2017

Nutrition Disaster Preparation Checklist

❑ Intravenous (IV) access

❑ Flushes (saline and/or heparin)

❑ Hand sanitizer

❑ Alcohol pads

❑ Batteries

❑ Filters and tubing (ex: Dial-A-Flow)

❑ Pre-mixed commercial PN (Clinimix® or Kabiven®)

❑ Normal saline (extended shelf life at room temperature)

Fig. 27.2 Nutrition checklist for disasters

Humanitarian Aid in Sudden Onset and Progressive Disasters

28

Asaf Kedar

Disasters are becoming more frequent as demonstrated in Fig. 28.1.

Humanitarian aid may be defined as assisting people in need, usually in a disaster area, with materials, logistics, and specialized skills. There are several agencies worldwide that have the ability to perform this mission. In general, external aid may be of great value until local infrastructure is restored to a point that it can be functional. However, it can be a burden if not done properly.

Images surfacing from disaster areas will always focus on the most visible effects of the incident and may not reflect the actual need for assistance.

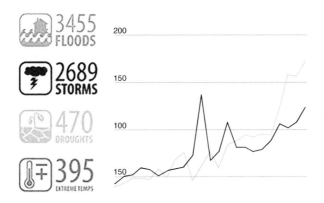

Fig. 28.1 Illustration of the rise of climate-related disasters around the world. Source: The United Nations Office for Disaster Risk Reduction, Created on 13 June 2012

A. Kedar
Jackson Memorial Hospital, University of Miami Miller School of Medicine, DeWitt Daughtry Family Department of Surgery, Division of Trauma/Critical Care/Burns, Miami, FL, USA

© Springer Nature Switzerland AG 2019
M. Lynn et al. (eds.), *Disasters and Mass Casualty Incidents*,
https://doi.org/10.1007/978-3-319-97361-6_28

Example: Images of food shortage may reflect difficulties in distribution and not actual lack of food in the area. The difficulties in distribution may be due to multiple reasons:
- Blocked roads
- Lack of vehicles
- Lack of organization
- Lack of prioritization

Hence, prior to delivering humanitarian aid, it is critical to establish what is needed.

The need can be established by:
- Communicating with local authorities
- Communicating with coordinating agencies for humanitarian aid, such the UN Office for the Coordination of Humanitarian Affairs (OCHA), which carries out its coordination function primarily through Inter-Agency Standing Committee (IASC)
- Communicating with other humanitarian organization that already deployed to the area
- Sending a pioneer team to survey the need in the affected area

There are several types of disasters as discussed previously. Humanitarian aid needs to be tailored to the type of disaster.

Humanitarian aid can take many forms, some examples are:
- Search and rescue operations
- Emergency communication
- Mass feeding
- Providing clean water
- Providing shelter and repairing homes
- Health care (Fig. 28.2)
- Psychological care
- Farm animals and pet rescue and care
- Building barriers and sandbagging

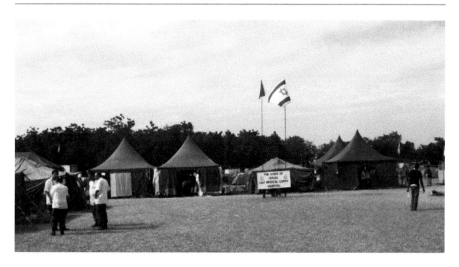

Fig. 28.2   Israeli field hospital in Haiti, 2010

Mental Health Support During and in the Aftermath of Disasters

29

Lior Lynn and Tanya L. Zakrison

As discussed previously, catastrophes can be diverse and range from natural sudden onset disasters such as hurricanes and earthquakes, to man-made sudden mass casualty incidents (SMCIs). Research shows that man-made SMCIs have a higher prevalence of posttraumatic stress disorder (PTSD) and other symptoms as compared to natural disasters. SMCIs can be overwhelming, devastating, and life threatening for individuals directly affected and others that are indirectly affected. This is true for survivors of SMCIs, the families of survivors, or communities that are grieving, living in fear, or attempting to rebuild. Handling the mental health of each of these groups is vital, as well as knowing how to differentiate between the processing abilities of these events by survivors at the extremes of age, such as the elderly and in particular, children. Specific to youngsters, it is important to identify their developmental stage, the cultural context, and atmosphere in which the children grow up and live, and the type of event (acute vs. chronic; natural vs. man-made). These variables are important for mental health-care providers when protecting against psychological harm.

Other persons impacted by MCIs include rescue and health-care professionals who are frequently exposed to these traumatic events. Nonetheless, there is a general way to prepare, manage, and treat those affected by mass casualty incidents, from a mental health perspective, to mitigate ongoing psychological trauma from such events.

How people react to psychological trauma depends on many factors as follows:
- Age: children of different age groups react differently
- Nature and severity of the event(s)

L. Lynn (✉)
Lynn Therapy, LLC, Pembroke Pines, FL, USA

T. L. Zakrison
University of Miami Miller School of Medicine, Jackson Memorial Hospital,
Department of Surgery, Miami, FL, USA

© Springer Nature Switzerland AG 2019
M. Lynn et al. (eds.), *Disasters and Mass Casualty Incidents*,
https://doi.org/10.1007/978-3-319-97361-6_29

- Prior experience with distressing events
- Preexisting support
- Prior physical health
- Personal and family history of mental health problems
- Cultural background and traditions

The most common diagnoses after a MCI, for both adults and children, include:
- Posttraumatic stress disorder (PTSD)
  - Experience with suicide bombers in Israel showed a prevalence of 5–10% of PTSD among survivors. In the aftermath of the Gulf War in 1991, about 40% of Israeli citizens experienced symptoms of PTSD, related to the Scud missiles attacks on their cities.
  - Symptoms and signs differ among adults and children and across genders. For example, anger and aggression, frequently misdiagnosed as a conduct disorder, may be the first sign of PTSD in boys and young men who have been survivors of a SMCI. Children struggling with PTSD are also often diagnosed with ADHD, as symptoms tend to be very similar, and traumas may be overlooked. It is important to know the different symptoms and signs for the gender or age group at hand, to avoid missing an opportunity for diagnosis and intervention.
- Acute stress disorder
  - It should be emphasized that it would be difficult to distinguish between a normal stress reaction and acute stress disorder (with the increased risk of developing PTSD) until 10 to 14 days after the incident.
- Adjustment disorder
- Depression, also presenting as anger in children and men
- Behavioral difficulties/regression in behavior or development
- Survivors guilt: feelings of guilt for surviving while others are injured or dead
- Poor concentration
- Restlessness
- Hyperactivity
- Difficulties with emotional regulation
- Avoidance of places/topics
- Panic disorder
- Fear
- Anxiety disorders: Separation anxiety, stranger anxiety for children
- Withdrawal
- Sleep problems.
- Dissociation/hallucinations

Screening for such psychopathology in the short and long term for both adults and children post-SMCIs is, thus, crucial to allow for appropriate treatment and a return to baseline function.

Planning and Preparation Before Progressive Disasters (e.g. Hurricanes)

If there is time to prepare, it is important to discuss and provide resources to people who will be affected by the incident:
- Provide tools for adults to handle their stress
- Provide children with a sense of safety, exploring ways to talk to them about what is going to happen, while establishing resources during and after the event, such as shelters, food resources, and counseling centers.
- Encourage adults to have their children be part of the preparation process. This may reduce negative psychological outcomes by making children feel safer and empowering them
- Facilitate and encourage discussions at schools, about emotional responses regarding the event that is about to happen
- Provide children with psychoeducation and coping strategies to use before and during the event.
- Provide children with supportive counseling to those who are feeling anxious during the preparation stage

Mental Health Response After a Disaster or SMCI

This is the most important time to intervene psychologically for those survivors directly affected, and those who are indirectly affected a SMCI. Some disasters can leave people stranded for hours, days, weeks (hurricanes, floods, earthquakes), and loved ones may be separated from one another without knowing of each other's fate. Many may lose their homes, personal possessions, and may have to rebuild their lives from the ground up. This is why it is so important to work with the families and communities that are affected and not only with the injured of these disasters.

Designated lead agencies have very few protocols for crisis situation to provide extensive psychological support. In some situations, provincial, regional, or state-level mental health departments may lead. In others, the responsibility may fall on municipal care providers.

There is, however, the concept of providing short-term psychological first aid (PFA). PFA actions is designed to meet the immediate practical needs of survivors, not to offer extensive psychological treatment. There is a previously established and freely available "Psychological First Aid guide for field workers" developed by the World Health Organization, available in 23 languages. Their guide covers psychological first aid which involves humane, supportive, and practical help to fellow human beings suffering serious crisis events. It is written for people in a position to help others who have experienced an extremely distressing event. It gives a framework for supporting people in ways that respect their dignity, culture, and abilities.

Below are the eight core actions outlined in PFA:

- Contact and engagement. Goal: Respond to contacts initiated by affected persons or initiate contacts in a nonintrusive, compassionate, and helpful manner
- Safety and comfort. Goal: Enhance immediate and ongoing safety and provide physical and emotional comfort
- Stabilization (if necessary). Goal: To calm and orient emotionally overwhelmed/distraught survivors
- Information gathering: current needs and concerns. Goal: Identify immediate needs and concerns, gather additional information, and tailor psychological first aid interventions
- Practical assistance. Goal: To offer practical help to the survivor in addressing immediate needs and concerns
- Connection with social supports. Goal: To reduce distress by helping structure opportunities for contacts with primary support persons or other sources of support, including family members, friends, and community helping resources
- Information on coping support. Goal: To provide the individual with information (including education about stress reactions and coping) that may help him or her deal with the event and its aftermath
- Linkage with collaborative services. Goal: To link survivors with services and inform them about services that may be needed in the future

According to various studies and the consensus of many crisis helpers, PFA involves factors that seem to be most helpful for long-term recovery. These include the following:

- Feeling safe, connected to others, calm, and hopeful
- Having access to social, physical, and emotional support
- Feeling able to help themselves as individuals and communities

Many survivors will not use or may not know of mental health services, and so it is vital to provide the affected community with knowledge of available services, using communication through mass media, or by organizing community outreach in municipal centers, if mass media is unavailable. Allowing online counseling services, if available, can also help reach out to more people who may not want to come face to face with psychological support providers due to stigma, or lack of transportation. Providing presentations in community centers, schools, religious centers, and other communal areas can also help gain access to communities that may not reach out for help otherwise or may not have access to internet resources or electricity altogether.

Allowing mental health volunteers to register to help the community online, if available, provided proof of licensure, can also allow a wide range of counselors to help after such mass disasters, as many times counselors are limited and are in need. In the event that online help is not applicable, having local centers where mental health volunteers can register and provide outreach services may be useful.

Methods

Crisis counseling is usually limited to 1–3 sessions and is provided by licensed clinicians who are trained in trauma and crises management counseling. As opposed to PFA, crisis counselors are trained professionals who provide psychoeducation to help understand PTSD and/or other symptoms that may arise (instead of recognizing it as a failure or weakness). Counselors also provide appropriate ways to cope and resources available in the community, emphasize the use of social support, and identify individuals that should seek further treatment by psychotherapists, psychiatric professionals, or community-based support groups.

Some interventions that tend to be used during crisis counseling include, but are not limited to:
- Supportive counseling
- Cognitive behavioral therapy (CBT)
- Brief trauma grief focused psychotherapy
- Play therapy: For children – notice repetitive play, reenactment
- Group therapy
- Community-based group therapy for adults and children

Checklist of how to prepare for a disaster:
- Develop a group of local mental health professionals for a crisis response
- Plan for shelters and counseling centers for families affected
- Access to resources that can be provided online, if available, for those affected
- Define who is in charge of the local mental health crisis management
- Interact with the media and provide resources and information to the public
- Establish a mental health phone hotline open for the public, as well as online counseling services, if applicable

Teamwork During Mass Casualty Incidents and Disasters

30

Kenneth Stahl

Teamwork is an essential and integral part of the successful management of sudden mass casualty incidents (SMCIs) and disasters. Teams are groups of people with similar objectives but differing levels of expertise and skills. Therefore, team leadership skills are also essential. Teams are made up of many people, but teamwork itself is an individual skill. During a SMCI, the formation of an effective team unit is complicated by the emergency nature of the incident and confounded by the confusion and chaos that these incidents generate. For these reasons, educating teams regarding their expected knowledge and skills are critical elements of planning for SMCIs. Developing and practicing team skills are a mandatory part of every mass casualty drill.

Effective teams:
- Function efficiently in high stress and time restricted environments.
- Recognize potential problems or dangerous circumstances and adjust their strategies accordingly.
- High-level performing teams exhibit a sense of collective efficacy and recognize that they are dependent upon each other to solve challenges when responding to SMCI's.
- Are dynamic.
- Optimize resource utilization.
- Engage in self-correction.
- Compensate for each other by providing backup behaviors and reallocate functions as necessary.
- Good teamwork establishes and maintains group and individual situational awareness and provides mutual support. Key benefits of good teamwork include added knowledge and expertise available to confront situations with synergy of ideas and skills so that the combined expertise of the team is greater than any

K. Stahl
University of Miami Miller School of Medicine, Jackson Memorial Hospital,
Department of Surgery, Miami, FL, USA
e-mail: kstahl@med.miami.edu

© Springer Nature Switzerland AG 2019
M. Lynn et al. (eds.), *Disasters and Mass Casualty Incidents*,
https://doi.org/10.1007/978-3-319-97361-6_30

individual. This synthesis of ideas and skills make multiple options available that a rapidly changing SMCI requires. Good teams create a "big picture" of situational awareness together and share information, perceptions, and ideas to keep everyone ahead of the evolving incident.

The characteristics of effective team formation and teamwork that should be incorporated in every mass casualty drill and incident management include:
- Establish the safety of the mass casualty environment to optimize team function.
- Nominate and establish the team leader.
- Rapid assessment of available potential team members including medical personnel, military, and police personnel, able-bodied civilians.
- Assemble team and assign roles.
- Team leader coordinates activities and assigns appropriate tasks to each team participant.
- Establish rapid and accurate communications so that decisions are clearly stated and acknowledged.
- Triage injured patients and prioritize tasks to avoid task overload.
- Maintain and control and safety of an operational environment.
- Assure team members are able to speak up and state their information in appropriate, assertive, persistent, and timely manner.

Effective leadership and supervision are crucial parts of team dynamics that should be repeatedly emphasized in mass casualty practice drills. Mass casualty team leaders perform the following key functions (Fig. 30.1):
- Provide strategic direction and backup
- Make appropriate assignments to team members based on skill and proficiency
- Monitor the performance of the team as a group and each individual team member
- Provide encouragement and assistance so team maintains best performance
- Assure all assignments have been carried out
- Maintain adaptability and flexibility
- Manage uncertain and urgent situations
- Share and disseminate accurate information and knowledge
- Avoid rumors and panic
- Assure accurate communication and close communication loop on all instructions and tasks

As a member of a mass casualty team, each participant also needs to practice good team skills. This includes:
- Listening carefully to the team leader instructions
- Promptly carry out assigned tasks
- Monitor other team members and offer assistance as needed so they can accomplish assigned tasks

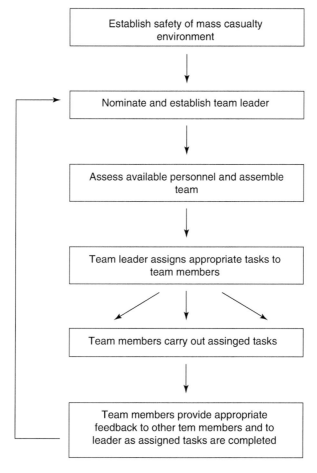

Fig. 30.1 Teamwork and team skills algorithm in Mass Casualty Management

- Provide accurate, timely, and assertive yet respectful feedback to the team leader and other team members
- Observe other team members for task overload, fatigue, and stress
- Maintain and contribute to team situational awareness
- Maintain vigilance for changing situations and additional safety risks
- Report any changes, progress and failures to the team leader

In summary, basic team skills and safety tools used in the management of trauma and critical care patients may be adapted for use in a SMCI.

Suggested Reading List

1. Active shooter incidents in the United States from 2000–2016, U.S. Department of Justice, Federal Bureau of Investigation; 2016. FBI.gov.
2. Adini B, Peleg K. On constant alert: lessons to be learned from Israel's emergency response to mass-casualty terrorism incidents. Health Aff (Millwood). 2013;32(12):2179–85. https://doi.org/10.1377/hlthaff.2013.0956.
3. Adini B, Goldberg A, Cohen R, Laor D, Bar-Dayan Y. Evidence-based support for the all-hazards approach to emergency preparedness. Isr J Health Policy Res. 2012;1(1):40. https://doi.org/10.1186/2045-4015-1-40.
4. Aharonson-Daniel L, Klein Y, Peleg K, ITG. Suicide bombers form a new injury profile. Ann Surg. 2006;244(6):1018–23.
5. AMA Journal of Ethics. Disaster and mass casualty triage. journalofethics.ama-assn.org/2010/06/cprl1-1006.html.
6. American College of Surgeons Bulleting Supplement. September 2015. Lakstein D, Blumenfeld A, Sokolov T, Lin G, Bssorai R, Lynn M, Ben-Abraham R. Tourniquets for hemorrhage control on the battlefield: a 4 year accumulated experience. J Trauma. 2003;54(5 Suppl):S221–5.
7. Arnold JL, Dembry LM, Tsai MC, Dainiak N, Rodoplu U, Schonfeld DJ, Paturas J, Cannon C, Selig S. Recommended modifications and applications of the Hospital Emergency Incident Command System for hospital emergency management. Prehosp Disaster Med. 2005;20(5):290–300.
8. Barbier EB. Policy: Hurricane Katrina's lessons for the world. Nature. 2015;524(7565):285–7.
9. Baxter PJ, Jenkins S, Seswandhana R, Komorowski JC, Dunn K, Purser D, Voight B, Shelley I. Human survival in volcanic eruptions: Thermal injuries in pyroclastic surges, their causes, prognosis and emergency management. Burns. 2017;43(5):1051–69.
10. Beekley AC, Sebesta JA, Blackbourne LH, Herbert GS, Kauvar DS, Baer DG, Walters TJ, Mullenix PS, Holcomb JB, 31st Combat Support Hospital Research Group. Prehospital tourniquet use in Operation Iraqi Freedom: effect on hemorrhage control and outcomes. J Trauma. 2008;64(2 Suppl):S28–37.
11. Bloch YH, Schwartz D, Pinkert M, Blumenfeld A, Avinoam S, Hevion G, Oren M, Goldberg A, Levi Y, Bar-Dayan Y. Distribution of casualties in a mass-casualty incident with three local hospitals in the periphery of a densely populated area: lessons learned from the medical management of a terrorist attack. Prehosp Disaster Med. 2007;22(3):186–92.
12. Brodie S, Hodgetts TJ, Ollerton J, McLeod J, Lambert P, Mahoney P. Tourniquet use in combat trauma: U.K. military experience. J Army Med Corps. 2007;153:310–3.
13. Cahill J, IMR Group Inc. When time stops: family support after a mass-casualty incident. 2010, June 16. Retrieved April 16, 2018, from https://www.domesticpreparedness.com/healthcare/when-time-stops-family-support-after-a-mass-casualty-incident/.
14. Carlsen HK, Hauksdottir A, Valdimarsdottir UA, Gíslason T, Einarsdottir G, Runolfsson H, Briem H, Finnbjornsdottir RG, Gudmundsson S, Kolbeinsson TB, Thorsteinsson T, Pétursdóttir

G. Health effects following the Eyjafjallajokull volcanic eruption: a cohort study. BMJ Open. 2012;2(6):e001851.

15. Cheatham ML, Smith CP, Ibrahim JA, Havron WS, Lube MW, Levy MS, Ono SK. Orlando Regional Medical Center responds to Pulse nightclub shooting. Bull Am Coll Surg. 2016;101(11):12–9.

16. Cherry K. How crisis counseling can help you cope with traumatic events. 2017. Retrieved April 16, 2018, from https://www.verywellmind.com/what-is-crisis-counseling-2795060.

17. Doocy S, Daniels A, Dooling S, Gorokhovich Y. The human impact of volcanoes: a historical review of events 1900–2009 and systematic literature review. PLoS Curr. 2013;16:5.

18. Einav S, Feigenberg Z, Weissman C, Zaichik D, Caspi G, Kotler D, Freund HR. Evacuation priorities in mass casualty terror-related events: implications for contingency planning. Ann Surg. 2004;239(3):304–10.

19. Gard BA, Ruzek JI. Community mental health response to crisis. J Clin Psychol. 2006;62(8):1029–41.

20. Get your kids on your team! n.d. Retrieved from https://www.ready.gov/kids/parents.

21. Goralnick E, Halpern P, Loo S, Gates J, Biddinger P, Fisher J, Velmahos G, Chung S, Mooney D, Brown C, Barnewolt B, Burke P, Gupta A, Ulrich A, Hojman H, McNulty E, Dorn B, Marcus L, Peleg K. Leadership during the Boston Marathon bombings: a qualitative after-action review. Disaster Med Public Health Prep. 2015;22:1–7. [Epub ahead of print].

22. Guidance on dealing with fatalities in emergencies, UK Home Office Communication Directorate 2004. https://assets.publishing.service.gov.uk/government/uploads/system/uploads/attachment_data/file/61191/fatalities.pdf.

23. Guidelines for the operation of burn centers (pp. 79–86). Resources for Optimal Care of the Injured Patient 2006, Committee on Trauma, American College of Surgeons.

24. Gupta BD. Mass disasters: a preparedness plan book with particular emphasis on mortuary services. JIAFM. 2004;26(2):0971-0973. ISSN 0971-0973.

25. Hafiz SCB, Attiyat M, Sussman M, Rattan R, Zakrison T, Garcia G, Marttos A, Lieberman H, Kaufman J, Hart V, Ruiz G, Schulman C, Pizano L, Byers P, Ginzburg E, Namias N, Pust G. In the eye of hurricane irma – traumatic injuries secondary to hurricane impact. Abstract, Flroia Committee on Trauma Meeting, Orladno, Florida; 2018.

26. Halpern P, Tsai MC, Arnold JL, Stok E, Ersoy G. Mass-casualty, terrorist bombings: implications for emergency department and hospital emergency response (Part II). Prehosp Disaster Med. 2003;18(3):235–41.

27. Hirshberg A, Scott BG, Granchi T, Wall MJ Jr, Mattox KL, Stein M. How does casualty load affect trauma care in urban bombing incidents? A quantitative analysis. J Trauma. 2005;58(4):686–93; discussion 694–5(ISSN: 0022-5282).

28. Jaffe DH, Peleg K, Israel Trauma Group. Terror explosive injuries: a comparison of children, adolescents, and adults. Ann Surg. 2010;251(1):138–43. https://doi.org/10.1097/SLA.0b013e3181b5d7ab.

29. Jensen J, Thompson S. The Incident Command System: a literature review. Disasters. 2015. https://doi.org/10.1111/disa.12135. [Epub ahead of print].

30. Kar N. Psychological impact of disasters on children: Review of assessment and interventions. World J Pediatr. 2009;5(1):5–11.

31. Kellermann AL, Peleg K. Lessons from Boston. N Engl J Med. 2013;368(21):1956–7. https://doi.org/10.1056/NEJMp1305304. Epub 2013 Apr 24.

32. Klima DA, Seiler SH, Peterson JB, Christmas AB, Green JM, Fleming G, et al. Full-scale regional exercises: closing the gaps in disaster preparedness. J Trauma Acute Care Surg. 2012;73(3):592–7; discussion 7–8.

33. Kluger Y, Peleg K, Daniel-Aharonson L, Mayo A, Israeli Trauma Group. The special injury pattern in terrorist bombings. J Am Coll Surg. 2004;199(6):875–9.

34. Kosashvili Y, Aharonson-Daniel L, Peleg K, Horowitz A, Laor D, Blumenfeld A. Israeli hospital preparedness for terrorism-related multiple casualty incidents: can the surge capacity and injury severity distribution be better predicted? Injury. 2009;40(7):727–31. https://doi.org/10.1016/j.injury.2008.11.010. Epub 2009 Apr 23.

35. Kragh JF Jr, Walters TJ, Baer DG, et al. Survival with emergency tourniquet use to stop bleeding in major limb trauma. Ann Surg. 2009;249(1):1–7.

36. Landman A, Teich JM, Pruitt P, Moore SE, Theriault J, Dorisca E, Harris S, Crim H, Lurie N, Goralnick E. The Boston Marathon bombings mass casualty incident: one emergency department's information systems challenges and opportunities. Ann Emerg Med. 2015;66(1):51–9. https://doi.org/10.1016/j.annemergmed.2014.06.009. Epub 2014 Jul 3.

37. Levi L, Michaelson M, Admi H, Bregman D, Bar-Nahor R. National strategy for mass casualty situations and its effects on the hospital. Prehosp Disaster Med. 2002;17(1):12–6. Review.

38. Li HL, Tang WJ, Ma YK, Jia JM, Dang RL, Qiu EC. Emergency response to nuclear, biological and chemical incidents: challenges and countermeasures. Mil Med Res. 2015;2:19. https://doi.org/10.1186/s40779-015-0044-3. eCollection 2015.

39. Lynn M, Gurr D, Memon A, Kaliff J. Management of conventional mass casualty incidents: ten commandments for hospital planning. J Burn Care Res. 2006;27(5):649–58.

40. Michaelson M, Reis ND. Crush injury–crush syndrome. Unfallchirurg. 1988;91(7):330–2. Review. No abstract available.

41. Michaelson M, Taitelman U, Bursztein S. Management of crush syndrome. Resuscitation. 1984;12(2):141–6.

42. Morgan O. Infectious disease risks from dead bodies following natural disasters. Rev Panam Salud Publica. 2004;15(5):307–12.

43. NASP School Safety and Crisis Response Committee. Recovery from large-scale crises: guidelines for school administrators and crisis teams. Bethesda: National Association of School Psychologists; 2018.

44. NASP: The National Association of School Psychologists, 2015. Ann Emerg Med. 1996;28(2):129–35.

45. National Child Traumatic Stress Network and National Center for PTSD. Psychological first aid field operation guide. 2nd ed; 2006. https://www.nctsn.org/resources/psychological-first-aid-pfa-field-operations-guide-without-appendices.

46. Noe RS, Schnall AH, Wolkin AF, Podgornik MN, Wood AD, Spears J, et al. Disaster-related injuries and illnesses treated by American Red Cross disaster health services during Hurricanes Gustav and Ike. South Med J. 2013;106(1):102–8.

47. O'Neill PA. The ABC's of disaster response. Scand J Surg. 2005;94(4):259–66.

48. Okumura T, Takasu N, Ishimatsu S, Miyanoki S, Mitsuhashi A, Kumada K, Tanaka K, Hinohara S. Report on 640 victims of the Tokyo subway sarin attack. Acad Emerg Med. 1998;5(6):618–24.

49. Peleg K. The danger of complacency – readiness and preparedness = effective outcomes. Ann Surg. 2014;260(6):967–8. https://doi.org/10.1097/SLA.0000000000000987.

50. Peleg K, Shenhar G. Did the U.S. Response to the marathon bombings help or harm security? FrontPublic Health. 2014;2:10. https://doi.org/10.3389/fpubh.2014.00010. eCollection 2014.

51. Peleg K, Michaelson M, Shapira SC, Aharonson-Daniel L. Principles of emergency management in disasters. Adv Ren Replace Ther. 2003;10(2):117–21. Review.

52. Peleg K, Jaffe DH, Israel Trauma Group. Are injuries from terror and war similar? A comparison study of civilians and soldiers. Ann Surg. 2010;252(2):363–9. https://doi.org/10.1097/SLA.0b013e3181e98588.

53. Pfefferbaum B, Pfefferbaum RL, Horn RL. Involving children in disaster risk reduction: The importance of participation. Eur J Psychotraumatol. 2018;9(Sup2):1425577. https://doi.org/10.1080/20008198.2018.1425577.

54. Pizzi MA. Hurricane Sandy, disaster preparedness, and the recovery model. Am J Occup Ther. 2015;69(4):6904250010p1–6904250010p10.

55. Raiter Y, Farfel A, Lehavi O, Goren OB, Shamiss A, Priel Z, Koren I, Davidson B, Schwartz D, Goldberg A, Bar-Dayan Y. Mass casualty incident management, triage, injury distribution of casualties and rate of arrival of casualties at the hospitals: lessons from a suicide bomber attack in downtown Tel Aviv. Emerg Med J. 2008;25(4):225–9. https://doi.org/10.1136/emj.2007.052399.

56. Schroll R, Smith A, NE MS Jr, et al. A multi-institutional analysis of prehospital tourniquet use. J Trauma Acute Care Surg. 2015;79(1):10–4.
57. Smith ER, Shapiro G, Sarani B. The profile of wounding in civilian public mass shooting fatalities. J Trauma Acute Care Surg. 2016;81(1):86–92.
58. Stein M, Hirschberg A. Medical consequences of terrorism. The conventional weapon threat. Surg Clin North Am. 1999;79(6):1537–52.
59. Teague DC. Mass casualties in the Oklahoma City bombing. Clin Orthop Relat Res. 2004;422:77–81.
60. The State of Florida fatality management response plan, Florida Medical Examiners Commission, Version 3.0; 2012. http://www.fdle.state.fl.us/MEC/Publications-and-Forms/Documents/MEC-Fl-Mass-Fatality-Plan-2018.aspx.
61. Tur-Kaspa I, Lev EI, Hendler I, Siebner R, Shapira Y, Shemer J. Preparing hospitals for toxicological mass casualties events. Crit Care Med. 1999;27(5):1004–8.
62. United States House of Representatives Committee on Oversight and Government Reform Majority Staff. Hospital emergency surge capacity: not ready for the "predictable surprise". 2008. https://www.hsdl.org/?view&did=485720.

Index

© Springer Nature Switzerland AG 2019
M. Lynn et al. (eds.), *Disasters and Mass Casualty Incidents*,
https://doi.org/10.1007/978-3-319-97361-6